Jenny Krutzinna • Luciano Floridi
Editors

The Ethics of Medical Data Donation

Editors
Jenny Krutzinna
Department of Administration and Organization Theory
University of Bergen
Bergen, Norway

Luciano Floridi
Oxford Internet Institute
University of Oxford
Oxford, UK

The Alan Turing Institute
London, UK

https://doi.org/10.1007/978-3-030-04363-6

Preface and Acknowledgments

New medical data is generated every second, adding to the source of potential "raw material" required for generating innovative and groundbreaking medical insights and expanding knowledge about health and well-being. For the first time in history, technologies exist that enable rapid and large-scale analysis of collected data, bringing the possibility of personalizing medicine within reach. Such positive prospects are countered by serious ethical, social, and legal challenges. Procedures for accessing medical data for research purposes, as well as for the reuse of medical data from clinical trials or studies, are in place and include safeguards to protect individual rights. However, no comprehensive scheme to donate one's medical data posthumously exists, with the consequence of depriving individuals of the opportunity to act according to their moral values and preventing valuable datasets from being used in scientific research for the promotion of the public good. While the debate around the use of big data in medicine is far from new, this volume is the first to address the ethical issues with regard to the use of medical data after death. It brings together academic experts from ethics, law, and medical sciences to address the challenges associated with medical data donation. It is the result of a project developed at the Digital Ethics Lab at the Oxford Internet Institute, University of Oxford, and funded by Microsoft Research.

We wish to thank the participants of the two workshops held in Oxford in October 2017 and April 2018 for their contributions to the discussion. Their input has been vital in developing the ideas for this volume and beyond. We would also like to thank the numerous peer reviewers that helped with the preparation of the individual chapters. Finally, we are grateful to Microsoft Research for the generous support of this project, without which it would not have been possible.

Bergen, Norway　　Jenny Krutzinna
Oxford, UK　　Luciano Floridi
London, UK

Contents

Contributors

Matthias Braun Department of Theology, Systematic Theology II (Ethics), Friedrich-Alexander-Universität Erlangen-Nürnberg, Erlangen, Germany

Peter Dabrock Department of Theology, Systematic Theology II (Ethics), Friedrich-Alexander-Universität Erlangen-Nürnberg, Erlangen, Germany

Luciano Floridi Oxford Internet Institute, University of Oxford, Oxford, UK

The Alan Turing Institute, London, UK

Bastian Greshake Tzovaras Lawrence Berkeley National Laboratory, Berkeley, CA, USA

Open Humans Foundation, Sanford, NC, USA

Ernst Hafen Institute of Molecular Systems Biology, ETH Zürich, Zürich, Switzerland

MIDATA Cooperative, Zürich, Switzerland

Edina Harbinja Aston University, Birmingham, UK

Patrik Hummel Department of Theology, Systematic Theology II (Ethics), Friedrich-Alexander-Universität Erlangen-Nürnberg, Erlangen, Germany

Kerina H. Jones Population Data Science, Swansea University Medical School, Swansea, UK

Jenny Krutzinna Department of Administration and Organization Theory, University of Bergen, Bergen, Norway

Philip J. Nickel Eindhoven University of Technology, Eindhoven, The Netherlands

Barbara Prainsack Department of Political Science, University of Vienna, Vienna, Austria

Department of Global Health & Social Medicine, King's College London, London, UK

David M. Shaw Institute for Biomedical Ethics, University of Basel, Basel, Switzerland

Care and Public Health Research Institute, Maastricht University, Maastricht, The Netherlands

Annie Sorbie School of Law, University of Edinburgh, Edinburgh, UK

Mason Institute for Medicine, Life Sciences and the Law, Edinburgh, UK

Mariarosaria Taddeo Oxford Internet Institute, University of Oxford, Oxford, UK

The Alan Turing Institute, London, UK

Athina Tzovara Helen Wills Neuroscience Institute, University of California, Berkeley, CA, USA

Chapter 1
Ethical Medical Data Donation: A Pressing Issue

Jenny Krutzinna and Luciano Floridi

Abstract While donation schemes with dedicated regulatory frameworks have made it relatively easy to donate blood, organs or tissue, it is virtually impossible to donate one's own medical data. The lack of appropriate framework to govern such data donation makes it practically difficult to give away one's data, even when this would be within the current limits of the law. Arguments for facilitation of such a process have been advanced but so far have not been implemented. Discussions on the ethics of using medical data tend to take a system-centric perspective and focus on what researchers and the health service may or may not do with data that are placed within their trust. Rarely, if ever, is the question of the data subjects preferences addressed beyond practical matters of obtaining valid consent. This constitutes an important omission in the ethical debate, which this volume seeks to address.

Keywords Data donation · Medical data ethics · Ethical code · Health records · Personal health data · Data philanthropy · Data ethics

1.1 Background

Donation has become a key concept in many areas of medicine, where it is now deeply engrained in everyday clinical practice, as well as in medical research. When physical donations are concerned, their importance of such medical donations is no

---

J. Krutzinna (✉)
Department of Administration and Organization Theory, University of Bergen, Bergen, Norway
e-mail: jenny.krutzinna@uib.no

L. Floridi
Oxford Internet Institute, University of Oxford, Oxford, UK

The Alan Turing Institute, London, UK
e-mail: luciano.floridi@oii.ox.ac.uk

J. Krutzinna, L. Floridi (eds.), *The Ethics of Medical Data Donation*, Philosophical Studies Series 137, https://doi.org/10.1007/978-3-030-04363-6_1

longer questioned, and increasingly medical governance systems are shifting from voluntary, opt-in models to opt-out schemes. Most recently, and in light of the introduction of the General Data Protection Regulation in Europe (GDPR), discussions have centered on the use of medical records for research purposes without the need for individual consent procedures, which are perceived as a significant obstacle to the advancement of medical insight and development of new treatments (Mann et al. 2016).

While donation schemes with dedicated regulatory frameworks have made it relatively easy to donate blood, organs or tissue, it is virtually impossible to donate one's own medical data. The lack of appropriate framework to govern such data donation makes it practically difficult to give away one's data, even when this would be within the current limits of the law. Arguments for facilitation of such a process have been advanced but so far have not been implemented (Shaw et al. 2016). Researchers are increasingly encouraged – and sometimes even required – to share their data in the name of science, and yet individuals cannot easily make their data available for scientific research purposes. This presents an ethically unjustifiable asymmetry in the biomedical research context: first, these datasets are of enormous importance for improvements in population health; and second, the difficulty infringes the autonomous decisions of many individuals who wish to contribute to the advancement of medical knowledge by making available their medical information.

Competing tensions on data control and ownership, respect of individual rights and consent, limited technical understanding, and the lack of adequate frameworks for coordination and ethical governance pose serious challenges to the donation of data and risk undermining its huge potential. The effect of the GDPR on medical data use is still uncertain, but some are concerned that it might be a serious impediment to scientific research and the re-use of data. Guidance to meet these challenges is urgently needed to ensure respect of users' individual rights and consent, foster transparency and trust, as well as harness the value of data to spur scientific research, public debate, private and public wellbeing.

The issue of systematically allowing private individuals to volunteer their medical data for research purposes has not yet been addressed in academic or popular literature, where emphasis has been placed mostly on data sharing between researchers, or on donations by private corporations in the context of data philanthropy (Taddeo 2016). However, empirical studies suggest that there is great willingness to allow medical data re-use on certain conditions, although medical donation schemes remain to this day largely limited to physical donations, such as organs, tissue or blood (Steinsbekk et al. 2013). There is significant scope to learn from posthumous physical donation schemes (Richardson and Hurwitz 1995), but the ethical and governance frameworks cannot be applied directly to data donation due to the specific characteristics of medical data. There is thus a need to develop a dedicated ethical code for posthumous data donation.

1.2 Current Debates

Discussions on the ethics of using medical data tend to take a system-centric perspective and focus on what researchers and the health service may or may not do with data that are placed within their trust. Rarely, if ever, is the question of the data subjects' preferences addressed beyond practical matters of obtaining valid consent. This constitutes an important omission in the ethical debate. The lack of comprehensive coverage of the topic of medical data donation has led the Digital Ethics Lab at the Oxford Internet Institute at the University of Oxford, to develop an ethical code for posthumous medical data donation (PMDD), in collaboration with Microsoft Research.

Two workshops were held in October 2017 and April 2018 to address the ethics of medical data donation. The aim of these workshops was to gather insight from academia, government, and industry in order to assess the risks and opportunities of PMDD. Participants came from diverse disciplines, and contributions covered topics related to the ethics of data donation, the legal and regulatory challenges posed by the donation of personal medical data, and current and future projects and collaborations in medical data donation.

Some key challenges were identified: trust, data quality, social values affecting the willingness to share data, impediments to corporate data sharing, and concerns around justice and inclusion. It was suggested to make health data sharing cases more tangible, by giving concrete examples of benefits for the stakeholders involved and practical information about the use and re-use of donated data. This was seen as potentially contributing to the removal of barriers to data donation by fostering a greater understanding of the process, including the risks involved. In addition, inclusion was mentioned as a key theme for further investigation, as current data donation projects such as the PGP UK are relatively exclusive, because they facilitate participation only by highly-educated, highly-engaged individuals ("Personal Genome Project: United Kingdom" 2018).

The ideas presented at the workshops and the discussions that ensued informed the development of the ethical code for PMDD presented in this volume. Many more ideas arose during the project and the workshops that could not be covered here. These included suggestions for next steps, including the extension of data donation to corporate data by means of data philanthropy schemes, and the addition of other data sources, such as health-related data collected by medical or lifestyle wearable devices. The latter raises important ethical issues beyond the scope of the present volume, such as the question of how to treat the digital remains of the dead (Öhman and Floridi 2018). Finally, the ethical code for PMDD proposed in this volume could eventually be extended to include donations made by living individuals, but for the reasons explained in the following chapters, we considered it ethically preferable to begin with deceased donations.

1.3 This Volume and Its Chapters

The book contains the proceedings of the two workshops held in Oxford, and some additional highly relevant contributions. It seeks to provide a timely analysis of the ethical use of existing personal medical data. The volume comprises four parts.

Part I seeks to conceptualise the ethics of medical data donation, by attempting to define what donation means in the context of data, and by identifying the key opportunities and ethical challenges of medical data donation.

Barbara Prainsack in "Data Donation: How to resist the iLeviathan" ascribes the distinctive characteristics of relationality, indirect reciprocity and simultaneity to data donation, as a specific type of transaction. She suggests that consideration of these characteristics could make data donation a strategy to counterbalance the overarching power of multinational enterprises. They have become 'a necessary monster' to which people submit their freedoms to in order to obtain other goods they consider essential.

In "Data Donation as Excercises of Sovereignty", Patrik Hummel, Matthias Braun and Peter Dabrock argue that data donations offer the potential to advance individual sovereignty, as they can generate social bonds, convey recognition and open up new options in social space. Articulating some of the difficulties associated with data donations, they call for thoughtful governance mechanisms and appropriate technological infrastructure design in response.

Philip J. Nickel in "The Ethics of Uncertainty for Data Subjects" discusses the practical uncertainties of modern data practices. He argues that significant endemic uncertainties undermine data subjects' interests in having grounds for trust in the institutions and organisations that control their data and proposes some possible ways of addressing this ethical problem.

Kerina H. Jones discusses the panoply of issues that may influence individuals' decisions with regard to data donation. In "Incongruities and Dilemmas in Data Donation: Juggling our 1s and 0s", she argues that although it would be unethical not to use donated medical data for the public good, it is crucial to acknowledge the conflicting beliefs and interests at play in data donation and which need to be carefully balanced.

In Part II, some of the key governance and regulatory challenges are discussed.

In her chapter, "Posthumous Medical Data Donation: The Case for a Regulatory Framework", Edina Harbinja outlines the most significant legal issues potentially affecting the donation of medical data after death and proposes how such a scheme would fit within the exiting legal framework governing health data.

Annie Sorbie in "Medical Data Donation, Consent and the Public Interest: A Gateway to Posthumous Data Use" suggests that in posthumous data donation, consent does not provide a 'magic bullet' and is only one aspect of a holistic governance regime. She argues that emphasis should be placed on the role of authorisation in this context.

Part III discusses the responsibility of all citizens to participate in medical data donation and provides some examples for implementation.

In "The Personal Data is Political", Bastian Greshake Tzovaras and Athina Tzovara use the examples of genetics and neuroscience to support their argument that in order to achieve truly personalized medicine, datasets need to be sufficiently diverse. They argue that this requires all of us to share our data for medical research purposes.

Ernst Hafen, in his chapter "Personal-Data Cooperatives – A New Data Governance Framework for Data Donations and Precision Health", explains one way in which this may be achieved. Calling for a more active role of citizens in the collection and management of personal data, he argues that data cooperatives are the perfect match for the challenges associated with the use of personal data, as they give democratic control to the citizen-owners.

In "Defining Data Donation After Death: Metadata, Directives, Guardians and the Road to Big Consent", David Shaw argues that given some ethical concerns, unconditional data donation may be premature and that a more cautious approach involving preference-setting through data advance directives and requiring family consent may be preferable as a first step.

Part IV concludes this volume with a discussion of the need for an ethical code for PMDD and the introduction of such a code.

In "Enabling Posthumous Medical Data Donation: A Plea for the Ethical Utilisation of Personal Health Data", Jenny Krutzinna, Mariarosaria Taddeo and Luciano Floridi argue that personal medical data should be made available for scientific research, by enabling and encouraging individuals to donate their medical records once deceased through PMDD. They stress the need to develop an ethical code for data donation to minimise the risks and conclude with the draft for such a code.

References

Mann, Sebastian Porsdam, Julian Savulescu, and Barbara J. Sahakian. 2016. Facilitating the ethical use of health data for the benefit of society: Electronic health records, consent and the duty of easy rescue. *Philosophical Transactions of the Royal Society A* 374 (2083): 20160130.

Öhman, Carl, and Luciano Floridi. 2018. An ethical framework for the digital afterlife industry. *Nature Human Behaviour* 2 (5): 318.

"Personal Genome Project: United Kingdom". 2018. https://www.personalgenomes.org.uk/.

Richardson, R., and B. Hurwitz. 1995. Donors' attitudes towards body donation for dissection. *The Lancet* 346 (8970): 277–279. https://doi.org/10.1016/S0140-6736(95)92166-4.

Shaw, David M., Juliane V. Gross, and Thomas C. Erren. 2016. Data donation after death. *EMBO Reports* 17 (1): 14–17. https://doi.org/10.15252/embr.201541802.

Steinsbekk, Kristin Solum, Lars Øystein Ursin, John-Arne Skolbekken, and Berge Solberg. 2013. We're not in it for the money—Lay people's moral intuitions on commercial use of 'their' biobank. *Medicine, Health Care and Philosophy* 16 (2): 151–162. https://doi.org/10.1007/s11019-011-9353-9.

Taddeo, Mariarosaria. 2016. Data philanthropy and the design of the infraethics for information societies. *Philosophical Transactions of the Royal Society A: Mathematical, Physical and Engineering Sciences* 374 (2083). https://doi.org/10.1098/rsta.2016.0113.

Part I
Conceptualising the Ethics of Medical Data Donation

Chapter 2
Data Donation: How to Resist the iLeviathan

Barbara Prainsack

Abstract Large corporations are attracting criticism for their quasi-monopolist role in the digital data domain. It has been argued that they are no longer regular market participants but have become *de facto* market regulators against whom public and civil society actors are powerless even when faced with stark ethical misconduct. Companies such as *Google*, *Amazon*, *Facebook*, and *Apple* (GAFA) have become a new Leviathan: a monster for which people give up freedoms in exchange for other goods that they consider essential. Data donation is a strategy that could, if certain conditions are met, help tackle the overarching power of multinational enterprises. I will propose that data donation, understood as a specific type of transaction, has three distinctive characteristics: relationality, indirect reciprocity and multiplicity. I suggest ways in which ethical and regulatory frameworks for data donation should consider these characteristics to ensure that data donations respond to the institutional and power relationships that digital data use is embedded in, that data donations contribute to the public good, and that they and protect the personal needs and interests of people involved in it.

Keywords Data governance · Data donation · Relational autonomy · Reciprocity · Solidarity

2.1 Data Use in the Era of GAFA

The French theorist Jean-Francois Lyotard, whose 1979 diagnosis of the end of the grand narratives is probably the most famous attempt to capture the meaning of the postmodern, was uncannily provident about the role that data would play in today's societies. Lyotard saw knowledge as having become a key factor in capitalist

B. Prainsack (✉)
Department of Political Science, University of Vienna, Vienna, Austria

Department of Global Health & Social Medicine, King's College London, London, UK
e-mail: barbara.prainsack@univie.ac.at; barbara.prainsack@kcl.ac.uk

J. Krutzinna, L. Floridi (eds.), *The Ethics of Medical Data Donation*,
Philosophical Studies Series 137, https://doi.org/10.1007/978-3-030-04363-6_2

accumulation processes.[1] The commercialisation of knowledge, he argued, results in shifts in how knowledge is valued, and how it shapes social and political institutions. Lyotard foresaw not only the decline of the privileged position of the state in controlling the production and distribution of knowledge,[2] but also, as political theorist Jeremy Gilbert put it,

> a decline in the prestige and potency of 'narrative' forms of knowledge which legitimate truth by reference to an over-arching story about the world, in favour of a *pragmatic* approach to knowledge which values 'truths' or fragments of knowledge solely on the basis of what instrumental or commercial effects they can produce (Gilbert 2014: 6. Original emphasis).

Paraphrasing Lyotard, the fragmentation of thick, narrative, and contextual knowledge into, quite literally, bits and pieces of data that are stripped of their social and political meaning is as one of the fundamental forms of the postmodern. Because not only information but also data are never 'raw', but they are embedded in relationships with the people and tools that created them (e.g. Gitelman 2013; Leonelli 2016), the practice of divesting data of their context is a central dynamic in this process.[3] The neutralising of data is done, for example, by tech companies, media outlets, and academics who treat data as a natural resource and compare it with water or with oil, that is, with something that nature gives us and that needs to be refined, filtered or bottled to be usable by humans (e.g. Puschmann and Burgess 2014; Anonymous 2017). By such a portrayal of data as natural resources these actors achieve three things: First, they place those who 'refine' the data–such as IT

---

[1] In Lyotard's own words:

> We may thus expect a thorough exteriorisation of knowledge with respect to the 'knower,' at whatever point he or she may occupy in the knowledge process. The old principle that the acquisition of knowledge is indissociable from the training (*Bildung*) of minds, or even of individuals, is becoming obsolete and will become ever more so. The relationships of the suppliers and users of knowledge to the knowledge they supply and use is now tending, and will increasingly tend, to assume the form already taken by the relationship of commodity producers and consumers to the commodities they produce and consume – that is, the form of value. Knowledge is and will be produced in order to be sold, it is and will be consumed in order to be valorised in a new production: in both cases, the goal is exchange (Lyotard 2004 [1979]: 4–5).

[2] Lyotard put it as follows: 'The notion that learning falls within the purview of the State, as the brain or mind of society, will become more and more outdated with the increasing strength of the opposing principle, according to which society exists and progresses only if the messages circulating within it are rich in information and easy to decode' (Lyotard 1979: 5).

[3] The historian Daniel Rosenberg is particularly eloquent in his description of the 'neutral' meaning of data in our societies: 'Data has no truth. Even today, when we speak of data, we make no assumptions at all about veracity. Electronic data, like the data of the early modern period, is given. It may be that the data we collect and transmit has no relation to truth or reality whatsoever beyond the reality that data helps us to construct. This fact is essential to our current usage. It was no less so in the early modern period; but in our age of communication, it is this rhetorical aspect of the term 'data' that has made it indispensable' (Rosenberg 2013: 37).

and consumer tech companies, governments, and other corporations–in a position where they have a moral right to profit from data because they supposedly built the infrastructures and tools to make data usable, and who mined or refined or packaged them for consumption. At the same time, by implying that data are a natural resource, they are rendering invisible the contributions that the people make who the data come from; as patients, as citizens, or as users of online services. Third, the allegedly de-politicised and de-contextualised nature of data portrays commercial corporations as fulfilling an important societal function, namely to create and analyse evidence about the world.

It is this allusion to the supposed public value of the data work they are doing that lets large multinational corporations who hold quasi-monopoly status get away with large-scale tax avoidance and questionable forms of data use. Some of the largest players in this landscape–including *Google*, *Amazon*, *Facebook* and *Apple* (GAFA)–have ceased to be market participants but become *de facto* market regulators, due to their immense size and influence (Pasquale 2017). They create facts on the ground that regulators need to catch up with, and they ensure that public authorities created legal frameworks and policies that facilitate the accumulation of power of GAFA. These policies include generous tax incentives, antitrust regulations that remain toothless against multinational tech corporations (e.g. Ip 2018), and data protection rules with unenforced sanctions or fines that remain below the pain threshold of multinational corporations (Golla 2017). The result is a profound power imbalance between those who use data and those from whom the data come, as well as the institutions that represent the interests of the latter (Pasquale 2017; see also van Dijck 2014; Zuboff 2015). GAFA have become a kind of new Leviathan – an *iLeviathan* (Prainsack 2018) – that people submit some of their natural freedoms to in order to receive something back that they consider essential; not physical security and the protection of their property, as was the case with the original, Hobbesian Leviathan, but the possibility to communicate across time and space, to buy goods in a faster and more convenient manner, and to use their time more effectively (for many, this is a necessary condition to be able to do all the other things they need to do to hold a job or two and run their families).

Responses to the profound power imbalances that data collection and use are embedded in the GAFA era have been manifold, in the public domain and within critical scholarship alike (e.g. Andrejevic 2014; Kaye et al. 2015; Brunton and Nissenbaum 2015; Pasquale 2017; Birkinbine 2018; see also Hummel et al. 2018). Many authors and initiatives seek to give people more control over how their own data are being used (e.g. Hafen et al. 2014); others focus on strengthening control and responsibility also at the collective level (e.g. Prainsack and Buyx 2016). Data donation could be an instrument that helps both ends: It could serve as an expression of a person's autonomy to decide what she wants to be done with her data, and as a commitment public value and collective control.

Before we proceed with the argument, there is one crucial question so solve: What does it mean to donate data?

2.2 What Does It Mean to Donate Data?

2.2.1 *Donation as a Relational Practice*

What is a donation? Legal definitions of the term all focus on the following elements: The owner of a thing transfers it to another person or entity without consideration of what she will receive in return. The latter aspect–that something is given without demanding something in return–tells us two things about donations: First, that they are outside of the commercial domain, meaning that no economic profit motive is attached to its transfer;[4] and second, that donations are not reciprocal. At least not in a direct and linear manner. Some definitions of donations suggest the word 'gift' as a synonym for donation to emphasise that both are embedded in networks of mutual moral and social obligations and subject to complex sets of rules. The behaviours of both gift-givers and gift-receivers are regulated by expectations about how and what to give and to receive, and they are sometimes faced with serious social repercussions if givers and receivers do not adhere to these unwritten rules (e.g. Caplow 1984; Carrier 1991; Bergquist and Ljungberg 2001; Zeitlyn 2003). In other words, gifts are indirectly reciprocal.

Why are these aspects important when thinking about data donations? First of all, they underscore the relational nature of donations. Their value, their consequences, and the practices of giving and receiving donations cannot be understood or assessed outside of the personal, social, and economic relations that they are embedded in. Definitions of donation express the relational nature of donations also by emphasising that donations are complete only once they have been received. My intention to donate something to you is not sufficient for the donation to materialise; you also need to receive it. And whether you will, or can, receive my intended donation, in turn, depends on a range of factors, such as: your trust in me (do you suspect my donation to be driven by questionable motives? Will it make you dependent on me? Or might the donation be harmful to you in any way?), your trust in institutions (is there somebody to turn to if something goes wrong?), possibly also on whether you feel you 'deserve' the donation, and on the various factors in your life that can foster or impede your ability to practically receive a donation. In the case of donations of money, it will be relevant whether you have a bank account. For an organ donation, it will be relevant whether or not you are eligible, and physically well enough, to undergo surgery. In other words, despite donation not being a commercial transaction, and despite their not being directly reciprocal in the sense that you do not need to give me something directly in return, my donation articulates, strengthens, or changes my relation to the person or entity that I donate something to, and vice versa.

---

[4]This does not preclude that the thing that is being donated has exchange value. For an excellent discussion of the distinction between commodification and commercialisation see Radin 1996.

2.2.2 *Can We Donate Data?*

Many of us will have something physical in mind when thinking of donations: books, organs, money. Money no longer sits in our pockets and wallets in the form of paper or coins, but, like books and organs, it is consumable and rivalrous: It can be 'used up', and the use of the good by one person affects the use of the good by others. If I donate money to an art school then I cannot give the same money to disaster relief. If I donate a kidney to one person, I cannot donate the same kidney to somebody else. Traditionally, donations have entailed that there is a consumable thing that is transferred from one entity to another. Can the same be said for data, and especially digital data?

I argued in another place that digital data are best described with the term multiplicity (Prainsack 2018). Multiplicity captures the characteristic of digital data of being able to be in more places than one at the same time, in leaving traces even when they are 'deleted', and of being able to be copied and used by several people at the same time, independent of what the others are doing.[5]

Returning to data donation, can we transfer something that is multiple? Can I 'donate' my medical records to a research project, or my DNA information to a biobank? I cannot do this in the sense that I transfer to somebody else a material thing that I then no longer have. In the case of data, if I allow researchers access to my medical records then I can still access them myself. So why do we not stick with the term data 'sharing', as this is what I am doing in the case of such 'donation'?

In the case of post-mortem use, there is a clear case to be made for the use of the term 'donation' over 'sharing' (Krutzinna et al. 2018), because 'sharing' implies joint use; if I share my car with you we can both use it, if we share a flat we both live in it. In the case of post-mortem data use, such a kind of sharing is not possible as the donor is no longer able to jointly use anything. But it is useful to use the term data donation also beyond the context of post-mortem donation: Whenever there is a non-commercial transfer of data from a living person to another, the term 'data donation' is arguably preferable to the very broad and unspecific 'data sharing'. The latter has been used to describe anything from agreeing to make one's medical information accessible to disease researchers to buying a DNA test online (Prainsack 2015). This lack of specificity muddles, rather than aids, the development of regulatory and ethical instruments in this field.

But to do justice to the specificity of the term data donation, as well as to the values enshrined in them, we need to consider a number of dimensions. *Relationality* is a characteristic of donation that tells us to be attentive to the relationships of

---

[5] Other terms that are often used to describe the nature of digital data, namely non-rivalry and non-depletability, assume that the value and integrity of data do not suffer from several people using them, and they cannot be 'used up'. Both of these assumptions are problematic, because the value of data can be affected by several people using them; think of proprietary information such search algorithms, or information on commercial mergers that are likely to affect stock prices.

both the giver and receiver of donations to their human, natural and artefactual environments, and to the needs and capabilities that emerge out of these relations. Attention to *indirect reciprocity* tells us to work towards frameworks that ensure that the relationship between givers and receivers is not starkly unbalanced in terms of the overall distribution of costs and benefits, duties and entitlements. Finally, the *multiplicity* of data–i.e. the fact that data can be, and often are, in different places at the same time–means that we can, and arguably need to, ask the question under what circumstances data donation should entail a transfer of rights to exclusive use, if at all.

2.3 Considerations for Frameworks for Data Donation

2.3.1 Relationality

I have argued that donations are relational in the sense that givers and receivers are connected through social, institutional, political, and economic relations. Moreover, not only are donors and receivers connected in this way, but also data themselves are relational. Despite the aforementioned efforts by some actors in our society to portray data as neutral evidence about the social and natural world that is out there independently of those who collect and analyse data (but that need to be made 'legible' through the valuable work of consumer tech companies), virtually all scholars and commentators who have been involved in, or studied, processes of data creation in practice agree that data in fact are inseparable and meaning-less if isolated from the humans and artefacts who created and sustained them (e.g. Leonelli 2016). As noted above, in contrast to what common comparisons of data with natural resources suggest, data are never 'raw' (Gitelman 2013).

Frameworks for data donations should take this relationality of people and data into consideration in at least two ways: first, by honouring the work that data donors–as patients, citizens, users of online services–have done to create the datasets in question; and second, by systematically considering the needs and interests of data donors and their significant others (family members, friends, and sometimes also non-human companions). Table 2.1 below summarises these concerns and includes questions that should be asked to ensure that these concerns are adequately considered in the creation of specific ethical and regulatory frameworks and instruments. To be clear, such consideration of the needs and interests of data donors (or those of their significant others, especially in the case of post-mortem donation) does not imply that data donors need to retain individual control over their data after the point of donation. Retaining individual control of the donor over data after the donation has completed would undermine the spirit of the very idea of data donation. Instead, a meaningful way of consideration of the needs of data donors and their significant others, and one that does not undercut the spirit of data donation, would be to call upon everybody using the data–clinicians,

Table 2.1 Considerations emerging from the relationality of data

Objective	Typical questions to be asked	Examples for implementation in ethical and regulatory instruments
Honour the work of data donors	What investments (in terms of time, money, training, community and infrastructure creation and maintenance) have (a) data donors and (b) communities and public actors made to create the dataset?	For example, acknowledgments of data donors, by name (if they have agreed to this), wherever appropriate, e.g. on a website, in publications for which their data have been used, etc.[a]
	What would a fair benefit for these actors to receive as an acknowledgement for their contributions?	
Consider the needs of data donors and their significant others	Should data donors retain access to their own individual-level data by default?	For example, data donors and their significant others could be offered to see copies of individual-level data that are donated. And data donors and significant others could be invited to opt into receiving updates on information obtained from their data (individual-level, actionable updates, is possible and appropriate, or alerts to aggregate findings or publications)
	Should significant others (biological relatives, or other named family members and friends) be told about findings stemming from the data donor's data that are likely to be significant and actionable in their own lives?	

[a]I am grateful to Jen Krutzinna for particularly helpful discussions on this point

researchers, or even the receivers of the donation–to ask questions about the value, benefits, and risks of data for different people, including the data donors. This means, for example, that if findings emerge from the data that are likely to make a significant difference in the data donor's or her family's life–such as serious and treatable health problems–the data donor or her family could be informed of this.[6] Another way to consider the needs of data donors would be to create processes and instruments to ensure that data donors retain access to their own data as it will continue to be their own health information (except in the case of post-mortem data donations, continued access by family members of the data donor could be considered). Given the fact that data can be used by several parties without necessarily detracting from the use value, this is typically not difficult to organise on the technical level.

[6]An important question, here, is under what conditions health information should be considered 'actionable' for the data donor and her family. Paperwork accompanying data donations should include information on the data donors' preferences in this request. Legislation should be in place to overrule the wishes of data donors who stated that they and their family members should not be contacted under any circumstances in cases where clinicians feel that not informing data donors (or their family members) of newly emerging information would put the donors or their family members in serious danger.

2.3.2 Indirect Reciprocity

I have noted that in contrast to other types of transactions that are characterised by direct reciprocity–that is, where one thing is exchanged for another in the same moment (a good or service for money, or goods for one another)–donations are not directly reciprocal. A transaction is not a donation if something is demanded in return. This does not mean, however, that donations take place in a social and political vacuum: Not only are givers and receivers connected through social, public, and economic environments and institutions, but in order for data donations to become a societal institution in itself that people trust, they need to be part of a system of indirect reciprocity. Potential and actual data donors need to know that the group that they are donating to, or that will benefit from their data–typically, the collective of people living in a specific country–will do give them something as well. Not directly, and not in the same instance as they decide to donate their data, but they will eventually provide assistance to them when they need it.

Such assistance could manifest itself in solidarity-based health insurance, where access to healthcare is not dependent on the ability to pay; or in progressive taxation of high salaries and transfer payments to those who do not have enough money to lead dignified lives. In the best of all worlds, all data donation frameworks are embedded in systems of such 'general' indirect reciprocity that ensure that people's fundamental needs and interests are met. But with regard to data donation specifically, indirect reciprocity–which is an inherently trust-building feature–should also manifest itself in institutions and instruments that ensure that data donors[7] who are harmed as a result of their donation receive support. Existing legal instruments are not sufficient for this purpose: Legal redress typically requires that the person who claims compensation for harm can prove that a specific action or omission by a specific actor causally led to the harm (or even that they broke a rule). In the digital era, however, where data are simultaneous and where proprietary algorithms and machine learning can make it impossible to trace how exactly data move through systems, legal instruments are out of reach for many who were harmed by data use. For this reason, Aisling McMahon, Alena Buyx and I have suggested the introduction of Harm Mitigation Bodies which would not require people to proof that a specific action or omission by a specific data user caused the harm. People appealing to Harm Mitigation Bodies would only need to show that the harm they experienced is plausibly connected to data use (McMahon et al. Under review). Harm Mitigation Bodies would judge the plausibility of the case and take any or all of the following three types of action: (1) feed information back to data controllers about the experienced harm and provide suggestions as to how such harm could be avoided in the future; (2) inform the person(s) experiencing the harm about what will be done to avoid such harms from occurring in the future, and issuing an apology if appropriate; (3) provide financial support. The first serves the purpose of creating a

[7] In the case of deceased donors, this extends also to significant others whom they leave behind.

Table 2.2 Three functions of Harm Mitigation Bodies in the context of data donation (McMahon et al. Under review)

Function 1	Function 2	Function 3
Collect information on the types of harm that occur as a result of data donations and feed this information back to data users	Inform those who experienced harm about what will be done to prevent such harm from occurring in the future	Provide financial support
	Issue apologies were appropriate	

record of the types of harms occurring from data use. Initiatives to create data harm records do thankfully exist already,[8] but Harm Mitigation Bodies would be in a position to create a systematic record of experienced harms. The importance of measures such as informing applicants about what will be done to avoid such harm in the future, and issuing apologies should not be underestimated. Empirical research in many contexts shows that people's experiences being 'seen' and acknowledged is a necessary step in the process of reconciliation and recovery from harm (e.g. Long and Brecke 2003; Staub 2006; Ramsbotham et al. 2011). Finally, regarding the third option of providing financial support, this would be an option of last resort if the person(s, or their family members) experienced significant and undue financial harm and there is no other source of financial support available. It should be emphasised here that the financial support function of Harm Mitigation Bodies are not meant to provide compensation or restitution, that is, these payments do not, and cannot, claim to be proportionate to the actual financial harm occurred. They are merely–but importantly–an instantiation of the societal commitment to support those who were harmed as a result of a prosocial practice, namely, donating their data. In another place we explain details as to how Harm Mitigation Bodies are governed, how they receive their funding, and on the basis of what criteria they make their decisions (McMahon et al. Under review) (Table 2.2).

We proposed that Harm Mitigation Bodies should be established at national levels and be subsidiary to legal remedies. They would be applicable to any instance of corporate data use, not limited to any specific domain or format of data 'sharing'. It would apply to harm resulting from deliberate and proactive data use (as in the case of data donation), or data use unbeknownst to the data subject (e.g. by using online services or when there is a legal basis for data use that does not require the person's consent). Harm mitigation is thus not only a design feature of data donation frameworks specifically but a necessary instrument of indirect reciprocity, which is a systemic property of the society that data donation frameworks are embedded in. It will help to ensure, on a systemic level, that the conditions under which people donate data are fair, and that data donation frameworks are trusted and trustworthy.

[8] E.g. https://datajusticelab.org/data-harm-record/

2.3.3 Multiplicity

The multiplicity of digital data, as noted above, means that data can be in several places at the same time, and that they typically leave traces where on their journeys (Leonelli 2016) throughout systems. In contrast to the paradigmatic example for things to be donated–money, clothes, or even organs–which are no longer available to the donor once the donation has been completed, data could, in theory, still be used by the donor and/or her significant others after the time of donation. I discussed some aspects of this above under the label of relationality earlier in this section, where I argued that the relationality of both people and data requires us to acknowledge the contributions of data donors and others to making the data available in the first place. I proposed that the most important way of acknowledging their 'data work' would be via considering the needs of data subjects and their significant others beyond the point of the donation. Here I wish to emphasise a related but different point, namely that the multiplicity of data raises the question whether the exclusive transfer of all rights pertaining to data is possible, and if it is possible, whether it is something that data donation *should* entail.

Let us start with the first part of the question, namely whether the exclusive transfer of all rights pertaining to data–including the right to use, destroy, and transfer ownership of the data–*can* be the subject of data donation. Again, if data were a clearly delineated material thing like a book or piece of clothing I could transfer all of these rights. This is the case because it is uncontested that property rights to books and clothes can be held and thus it is possible to transfer them. With regard to data, the situation is more complicated, because there is no consensus that property rights to data can be held. To put it very generally, in the United States and in areas influenced by U.S. law, there is the view that personal data can be governed by individual property regimes, which are often described as bundles of rights including the right to use the thing, to use it exclusively if one wishes, to earn income from the it, to transfer it to others, or to destroy it. In Europe and in areas influenced by European legal traditions, personal data tend to be seen as inalienable possessions of a person that are protected by human rights–such as privacy–and not by property rights. What might sound like a petty technical point signifies a large ideological difference: The purpose of property rights is to enable–and, as some would argue, to encourage–the *transfer* of goods, and thus the introduction of goods into markets and economic value chains. The European-style human rights approach, in contrast, treats data as something that have no price; as something that should not be commodified and commercialised (see also Purtova 2009, 2015; see also Prainsack 2018).

This means that if data donation takes place in a country that does not allow individual property rights to be held to personal data, the person owning (in a moral sense) her data cannot transfer property rights of data to another person because she does not hold them in the first place. We *can* allow others to use our data, but we cannot transfer the right to exclusive use, or the right to transfer legal ownership. In other words, as a data donor I can allow others to use my data, but I cannot transfer the *exclusive* right to these data. The multiplicity of digital data is the techno-material expression of the legal view of the non-transferability of exclusive rights data: I can allow others to use all of the data and information that I uploaded onto my social media sites but these can still be accessed by myself as well (and when I am dead, they can still be accessed by those I leave behind with my password).

If data donation takes place in a country that does treat personal data as individual property then I could, in theory, transfer the whole bundle of my property rights–and thus, exclusive control over my data–to others. Here, the multiplicity of digital data means that if I donate the data held in my digital home assistant, for example, to a university for their exclusive use, I would need to ensure that I no longer have access to the data in my home assistant myself (or my heirs and password holders after my death). The question here is whether such a scenario of transfer of right to exclusive use is practically enforceable, and if it is, if it is desirable.

2.4 Resisting the iLeviathan? Politicising the Ethics of Data Donation

In this paper, I explored the notion of data donation. I started by outlining the power relationships between citizens as data subjects on the one hand, and the corporations that use data on the other. I argued that both the political and, within it, the discursive economy that data use is embedded in, grants a number of moral and political rights to corporations that should belong to data subjects instead. I argued that data donation can be an instrument to change the political data economy for the better. Data donation, I argued, has three distinctive characteristics: relationality, indirect reciprocity, and multiplicity. For each of these characteristics I outlined what they mean for the design of ethical and regulatory instruments for data donation. With respect to relationality, I proposed that the consideration of the needs and interests of data donors (and their significant others) should remain an important concern also once a donation has been completed. The characteristic of indirect reciprocity mandates that we ensure that data donation frameworks are embedded in systems of structural mutual assistance and support. The characteristic of multiplicity–which, as noted, is not a property of the type of transaction but a property of digital data, which have the capacity to be in more than one place at the same time–raises the question of whether the transfer of exclusive control over data is possible, and if it is, whether it should be. I concluded that the answer to this question depends on whether or not we see personal data as something that can be governed by individual property rights. In countries where personal data are treated as an inalienable possession rather than individual property in the legal sense, it is not possible to transfer exclusive control over data because one does not have it in the first place. In such countries, data donations would amount to data donors consenting to some specific (but not unlimited) use rights by third parties. And even in countries where personal data are seen to be governed by individual property rights and the transfer of exclusive rights is legally possible, it is questionable whether the transfer of exclusive control is desirable, and practically feasible.

Last but not least, when designing ethical and legal frameworks for data donation, the consideration of the role that data donation should play in the political economy is of utmost importance. The notion of donation, as outlined aptly by Krutzinna, Taddeo and Floridi, treats the common good as a 'foundational ethical principle' (Krutzinna et al. 2018). The very idea of giving up control over one's data and allowing others to use them can be a symbol of trust in others (also beyond somebody's death), and an instance of solidarity. It can also be an expression of the data donor's autonomy: If I decide to donate my data then I am not leaving it up to 'the system' to decide, but I take an active decision that my data should create value for others too. This, however, will only work if the institutions that facilitate and govern data donation are trustworthy, and if they protect the needs and interests of data donors and data users both as individuals and as members of our society. If we want it to change our political economy for the better, then data donation could be a bridge between the individual and the public domain.

Acknowledgements I am grateful to Jen Krutzinna, Hendrik Wagenaar, and the anonymous reviewers for helpful comments on drafts of this paper, and the participants of the Data Donation workshop at the Oxford Internet Institute on 20 April 2018 for valuable discussions.

References

Andrejevic, M. 2014. Big data, big questions: The big data divide. *International Journal of Communication* 8: 1673–1689.

Anonymous. 2017. The world's most valuable resource is no longer oil, but data. *The Economist* (6 May). Available at: https://www.economist.com/news/leaders/21721656-data-economy-demands-new-approach-antitrust-rules-worlds-most-valuable-resource. Accessed 24 June 2018.

Bergquist, M., and J. Ljungberg. 2001. The power of gifts: Organizing social relationships in open source communities. *Information Systems Journal* 11 (4): 305–320.

Birkinbine, B.J. 2018. Commons praxis: Towards a critical political economy of the digital commons. *tripleC* 16 (1): 290–305.

Brunton, F., and H. Nissenbaum. 2015. *Obfuscation: A user's guide for privacy and protest*. Cambridge, MA: MIT Press.

Caplow, T. 1984. Rule enforcement without visible means: Christmas gift giving in Middletown. *American Journal of Sociology* 89 (6): 1306–1323.

Carrier, J. 1991. Gifts, commodities, and social relations: A Maussian view of exchange. *Sociological Forum* 6 (1): 119–136.

Gilbert, J. 2014. *Common ground: Democracy and collectivity in an age of individualism*. London: Pluto Press.

Gitelman, L. 2013. *Raw data is an oxymoron*. Cambridge, MA: MIT Press.

Golla, S.J. 2017. Is data protection law growing teeth: The current lack of sanctions in data protection law and administrative fines under the GDPR. *Journal of Intellectual Property, Information Technology and E-Commerce Law* 8: 70.

Hafen, E., D. Kossmann, and A. Brand. 2014. Health data cooperatives–citizen empowerment. *Methods of Information in Medicine* 53 (2): 82–86.

Hummel, P., M. Braun, and P. Dabrock. 2018. Data donation as exercises of sovereignty. In *The ethics of medical data donation*, ed. J. Krutzinna and L. Floridi. Springer.

Ip, G. 2018. The antitrust case against Facebook, Google and Amazon. *The Wall Street Journal* (16 Jan). Available at: https://www.wsj.com/articles/the-antitrust-case-against-facebook-google-amazon-and-apple-1516121561. Accessed 16 Aug 2018.

Kaye, J., E.A. Whitley, D. Lund, M. Mirroson, H. Teare, and K. Melham. 2015. Dynamic consent: A patient interface for twenty-first century research networks. *European Journal of Human Genetics* 23 (2): 141–146.

Krutzinna, Jenny, Mariarosaria Taddeo, and Luciano Floridi. 2018. Enabling posthumous medical data donation: A appeal for the ethical utilisation of personal health data. *Science and Engineering Ethics*. https://doi.org/10.1007/s11948-018-0067-8.

Leonelli, S. 2016. *Data-centric biology: A philosophical study*. Chicago: University of Chicago Press.

Long, W.J., and P. Brecke. 2003. *War and reconciliation: Reason and emotion in conflict resolution*. Cambridge, MA: MIT Press.

Lyotard, J.F. 2004 [1979]. *The postmodern condition: A report on knowledge*. (Translation from the French by Geoff Bennington and Brian Massumi) King's Lynn: Biddles.

McMahon, A., B. Buyx, and B. Prainsack. Under review. *Big data governance needs more collective agency: The role of harm mitigation in the governance of data use in medicine and beyond.*

Pasquale, F. 2017. From territorial to functional sovereignty: The case of Amazon. Law and Political Economy (6 December). *Law and Political Economy* blog. Available at: https://lpeblog.org/2017/12/06/from-territorial-to-functional-sovereignty-the-case-of-amazon/. Accessed 24 June 2018.

Prainsack, B. 2015. Why we should stop talking about data "sharing". Guest blog post on DNAdigest (1 December). Available at: http://dnadigest.org/why-we-should-stoptalking-about-data-sharing/. Accessed 24 June 2018.

———. 2018. *Logged out: Property, exclusion, and societal value in the digital data and information commons*. Under review.

Prainsack, B., and A. Buyx. 2016. Thinking ethical and regulatory frameworks in medicine from the perspective of solidarity on both sides of the Atlantic. *Theoretical Medicine and Bioethics* 37 (6): 489–501.

Purtova, N. 2009. Property rights in personal data: Learning from the American discourse. *Computer Law & Security Review* 25 (6): 507–521.

———. 2015. The illusion of personal data as no one's property. *Law, Innovation and Technology* 7 (1): 83–111.

Puschmann, C., and J. Burgess. 2014. Big data, big questions. Metaphors of big data. *International Journal of Communication* 8: 20.

Radin, M.J. 1996. *Contested commodities. The trouble with trade in sex, children, body parts, and other things*. Cambridge, MA: Harvard University Press.

Ramsbotham, O., T. Woodhouse, and H. Miall. 2011. *Contemporary conflict resolution*. Cambridge: Polity.

Rosenberg, D. 2013. Data before the fact. In *Raw data is an oxymoron*, ed. L. Gitelman, 15–40. Cambridge, MA: MIT Press.

Staub, E. 2006. Reconciliation after genocide, mass killing, or intractable conflict: Understanding the roots of violence, psychological recovery, and steps toward a general theory. *Political Psychology* 27 (6): 867–894.

van Dijck, Jose. 2014. Datafication, dataism and dataveillance: Big data between scientific paradigm and ideology. *Surveillance & Society* 12: 199–208.

Zeitlyn, D. 2003. Gift economies in the development of open source software: Anthropological reflections. *Research Policy* 32 (7): 1287–1291.

Zuboff, Shoshana. 2015. Big other: Surveillance capitalism and the prospects of an informal civilization. *Journal of Information Technology* 30: 75–89.

Chapter 3
Data Donations as Exercises of Sovereignty

Patrik Hummel, Matthias Braun, and Peter Dabrock

Abstract We propose that the notion of individual sovereignty encompasses more than having the power to exclude others from one's personal space. Instead, sovereignty is realized at least in part along outward-reaching, interactive and participatory dimensions. On the basis of reflections from gift theory, we argue that donations can generate social bonds, convey recognition and open up new options in social space. By virtue of these features, donations offer the potential to advance individual sovereignty. We go on to highlight distinctive benefits of *data* donations, before articulating several difficulties and puzzles: data donors are bound to have a limited grip on future uses of their data and the people affected by their decision to share. Further characteristic traits of data donations come from the invasive and comprehensive character of state-of-the-art data gathering and processing tools, and the fact that the relevant sense of data ownership is far from straightforward. In order to minimize tensions with negative, protective aspects of sovereignty, we argue that thoughtful mechanisms at the level of consent procedures, the representation of data subjects in governance structures, and organizational-level constraints are necessary. Along the way, we will devote particular attention to challenges and opportunities within big data contexts.

Keywords Digital sovereignty · Data donation · Data loan · Gift theory · Informational self-determination · Big data

P. Hummel (✉) · M. Braun · P. Dabrock
Department of Theology, Systematic Theology II (Ethics),
Friedrich-Alexander-Universität Erlangen-Nürnberg, Erlangen, Germany
e-mail: patrik.hummel@fau.de; matthias.braun@fau.de; peter.dabrock@fau.de

J. Krutzinna, L. Floridi (eds.), *The Ethics of Medical Data Donation*,
Philosophical Studies Series 137, https://doi.org/10.1007/978-3-030-04363-6_3

3.1 Introduction

Donations are common in health contexts. Crowdfunding calls through websites like GoFundMe in which patients rely on private donors to pay for unexpected medical expenses are familiar especially in the United States (Snyder 2016; Berliner and Kenworthy 2017). There are plenty of opportunities to help others not just by giving money, but also by giving parts of our bodies, such as organs or blood. We can give such parts or materials more or less directly to patients in need, or contribute samples to biobanks in which they feed into research, development, public health surveillance and other beneficial activities.

In these kinds of donations, the potential donor is in a position to seek and understand information about the need for her donation. Although some degree of uncertainty is often inevitable, she can learn about the features of potential recipients, the way in which her donation addresses a problem, and how her donation will be distributed. It is also quite straightforward what she is donating, e.g., an organ, blood, or a specimen. Moreover, the donor herself is carrying any inconveniences in connection with her donation, and burdensome effects on others are typically minimal or absent.

Databases are growing at breath-taking speeds, while tools and algorithms to process and interpret data become more powerful and sophisticated (Mayer-Schönberger and Cukier 2013; Murdoch and Detsky 2013; Raghupathi and Raghupathi 2014). Still, information that can feed into evidence bases is not always readily available. It needs to be discovered, harvested, shared, and analysed. In recent years, the roles individuals can play in data gathering processes have received increased attention. The widespread rollout of electronic health records has made it easier than ever to handle personal health data and opens up opportunities for sharing it in a variety of ways. By making their health data available, individuals can enable research and advance clinical progress (Nature Biotechnology 2015).

Two potential applications are the following. First, medical data can feed into research. By providing one's data for such purposes, one ideally provides researchers with the raw materials for discovering unforeseen correlations and helps to pave the way for new hypotheses, preventive actions, diagnostics, and treatments. One possible source for such data is direct-to-consumer genetic testing. For example, in 2014 the online networking service PatientsLikeMe launched its "Data For Good" campaign, which "underscores the power of donating health data to improve one's own condition, help others and change medicine" (PatientsLikeMe 2014). The campaign is motivated by survey data suggesting that "94 percent of American social media users agree with sharing their health data to help doctors improve care" (Grajales et al. 2014), provided their anonymity is secured. Further examples include the non-profit platform DNA.Land which calls for users to upload their genomic data in order to "enable scientists to make new discoveries" and to learn more about their genome (DNA.Land 2018). The open source website openSNP allows users to upload genetic information, including full genomes, which are then published under a Creative Commons Zero licence. The data can be freely copied, modified, distributed, and analysed for commercial and non-commercial purposes.

Second, an increasing number of clinical deep-learning-driven diagnostics and treatments rely on large amounts of patient data, cases, and background information. Data that is fed into such systems can guide a vast range of useful applications, e.g., the delineation of tumours in radiological images (Microsoft 2018) or therapeutic decision-making regarding metastatic breast cancer (Yang et al. 2016, 2017). Sharing one's personal health data for such purposes directly affects treatment options and prospects of present and future patients.

The question arises under which conditions applications like these can legitimately be based on donations of personal health data from individuals. The present paper argues that some of the most pressing challenges surrounding data donations are challenges about the data sovereignty of the donor. We begin by introducing the concept of data sovereignty (2.) and propose that it encompasses more than having the power to exclude others from one's personal space. Instead, it has a positive dimension as well. On the basis of reflections from gift theory, we propose that data donations can be exercises of positive data sovereignty. We go on to highlight potentials (3.) of data donations, before articulating several difficulties and puzzles that arise from the idea of donating personal health data (4.). We close with some suggestions on how sovereign data donations could be made possible in practice (5.). Along the way, we will devote particular attention to complications and opportunities within big data contexts.

Before we begin, a conceptual remark on the idea of donating one's personal health data is in order. While the concept of data sharing has received a lot of attention throughout the literature (e.g., Borgman 2012), the notion of data donation is relatively new and less widespread (e.g., Prainsack and Buyx 2017, ch. 5). Data sharing and data donation both involve the provision of access to data. In our view, they differ along at least two dimensions.

The first difference relates to exclusivity: if I *share* a good, I can still use at least a portion of it myself. If I *donate* something, typically the respective portion of the good is gone. Relative to ordinary language, it is thus somewhat surprising to speak of data *donations* insofar as the putative donor typically does not lose even a portion of her data when granting others access (see also Barbara Prainsack's contribution to this volume).

The second difference is motivational, and in our view provides an important reason to focus on data donations. Relative to ordinary language, the notion of donating more than the notion of mere sharing highlights the possibility of a particular kind of motivation for why we might give others access to our goods. When I *exchange* or *trade* something or a portion thereof, I expect a return. When I *gift* something, do I expect a return, too? As we will see in the following, this question is discussed controversially. What does seem to distinguish *gifting* from *exchanging* is that the former involves a symbolic dimension that the latter lacks. For this reason, the following discussion is driven by the suspicion that when reflecting upon data *donations*, we should be mindful of such symbolic aspects of granting others access to one's data.

3.2 Donations and Sovereignty

Many areas in the health sector anticipate progress and efficiency gains from increasingly powerful data gathering and processing tools. The hope is that such innovations will advance a range of activities such as public health surveillance, research and development, the provision of medical care and the design of health systems. While these prospects are intriguing, novel and ever more penetrative data-processing tools can leave individuals susceptible to risks of harm and prompt us to consider at what point disproportionate intrusions into the personal sphere begin—especially if highly intimate and sensitive information is being processed. Big data applications thus bring a number of ethical questions to the forefront (Nuffield Council on Bioethics 2015; Vayena et al. 2015; Mittelstadt and Floridi 2016; German Ethics Council 2017a, b), including how individuals can make autonomous choices about where their data goes and what is being done with it, while they shall be both beneficiaries *and* objects of investigation of data- and computation-intensive tools that promise to speed up and to enhance knowledge generation processes.

One up-and-coming concept in these discussions is the notion of data sovereignty. Although not used uniformly throughout the literature, the concept relates to issues of control about who can access and process data (Friedrichsen and Bisa 2016; De Mooy 2017; German Ethics Council 2017a, b). For example, data sovereignty is being discussed with regards to cloud computing, and refers to what is being undermined by uncertainty about which law applies to information stored in the cloud (De Filippi and McCarthy 2012). Commentators worry that governments which use cloud computing run the risk of compromising national sovereignty by conceding control over their data (Irion 2013). Some identify data sovereignty with the ability to geolocate data and to place it within the borders of a particular nation-state (Peterson et al. 2011). Only then is it possible for users to determine which privacy protections, intellectual property protections, and regulations apply, and which risks of legal and illegal access to data exist.

In the German media discourse, data sovereignty is occasionally being perceived as a threat to privacy and a "lobby notion" introduced by the data-processing industry to hollow out data protection standards (Krempl 2018). But quite the opposite is true. While data sovereignty does indeed rest on the conviction that traditional input-oriented data protection principles like data minimisation and purpose limitation are unsuitable in big data contexts (German Ethics Council 2017a, b), two important clarifications are in order. First, proponents of data sovereignty highlight its orientation towards informational self-determination, which involves the protection of a personal sphere of privacy that sets the stage for participation in the public sphere (Hornung and Schnabel 2009). Second, the notion of data sovereignty is driven by the conviction that claims and rights like those related to informational self-determination can only be realized against the backdrop of social contexts and structures in which they are articulated, recognized, and respected. Proponents of data sovereignty highlight that digitization has the potential to transform the social core in which articulations of these claims are always embedded. This is why it is inadequate to insist upon rigid, input-oriented data protection principles (Dabrock 2018). Instead, the focus must shift to the social transformations and tensions of digitization in which individuals should be put in a position to claim their right to informational self-determination reliably and robustly.

In the following, we shall not deny that sovereignty motivates negative and protective claims and rights related to the data subject's privacy (although cf. Goodman 2016, pp. 153–155). Instead, we will focus on the question whether the picture of sovereignty encompasses more than just the exclusion of others from one's personal information, and instead motivates claims of individuals to *share* rather than hold back their data.

In early modern political theory, sovereignty denotes absolute and unconditional power that is neither constrained by nor accountable to other powers. The notion became prominent after Bodin (1576) applied it to absolutist rulers in order to characterize their supreme authority. For Hobbes (1651), this authority is the result of a transfer of sovereignty from the people to the ruler. Other authors attributed sovereignty to nations, countries, or peoples. Sovereignty is typically indexed to a spatial or a substantive domain. The spatial domain is the territorial region which is subject to the sovereign's will. The substantive domain comprises the matters on which the sovereign is authoritative. Nevertheless, the claim to absolute power is one reason why the notion of sovereignty is sometimes being looked upon with uneasiness, and has led to controversies about whether the political sphere is framed fruitfully in terms of it. For example, Maritain (1951, ch. 2) worries that once the people transfer their power to the sovereign in Bodin's or Hobbes' model, their sovereignty is irretrievably lost. After having become the sovereign, the leader is free to determine the nature and boundaries of its power. Against this, one can invoke notions of legitimacy, and argue that sovereignty properly understood is undercut by certain claims to power and ways of ruling. The apparent sovereign becomes a despot if she is guided by arbitrariness and self-interest or proceeds without appropriate forms of recognition from the people she governs. Sovereignty, although *prima facie* a property of the authoritative individual, is not something which can simply be claimed and possessed independently of social or political embeddedness. It is something that is conferred upon the sovereign, a property that arises from its relation to those who are eventually subject to the sovereign power and recognize the sovereign as authoritative and legitimate.

The power of the sovereign goes hand in hand with the ability to constrain the power of others. Prior to early modern times, the historic function of the concept was not to entitle rulers to power, but to *delimit* the authority of worldly leaders. Sovereignty as unconstrained and absolute power was attributed to God in order to distinguish divine authority from claims of kings and emperors, and to *constrain* the claims to power of the latter. Modern ascriptions of sovereignty also have implications about negative freedom. For example, Mill argues that with regards to things which concern only the subject herself, she is entitled to absolute independence from interference by society: "[o]ver himself, over his own body and mind, the individual is sovereign" (Mill 1859, p. 224).

Nevertheless, sovereignty is not exhausted by negative claims. It can have *positive* implications about the space it determines as the domain of the sovereign. The sovereignty of a state is not exhausted by *external* sovereignty against outside interference. Instead, sovereignty has an *internal* dimension as well: within its territory the sovereign has the authority to govern according to her will. Similarly, Mill's individual who is the sovereign over her personal sphere is not merely entitled to the right and power to *exclude* others from her domain of sovereignty, but also to *operate* within this sphere—in Mill's case: to pursue her idea of the good life.

For either dimension, one important realizer of sovereignty is power. Sovereignty is being realized through the power to keep outsiders out of one's domain of sovereignty and to operate within this domain. This carries with it the constraint, criticism, and repudiation of claims to power of outsiders as well as those insiders who are subject to the sovereign. Again, this isn't crude and arbitrary power or force. Whether a claim to sovereign power is appropriate and legitimate depends on its content and the relationship between the putative sovereign and her claim's addressees. Negotiating sovereignty and its scope is a discoursive process to be carried out in dialogue with others and society.

When individuals pursue their idea of the good life, we should take note of the fact that this pursuit need not be exhausted by an atomistic sense of one's personal good. As Taylor (1985, p. 190) maintains: "Man is a social animal, indeed a political animal, because he is not self-sufficient alone, and in an important sense is not self-sufficient outside a polis." The sovereign individual's pursuit of the good life plausibly unfolds through social relations, embeddedness, and interactions. Crucial realizers of positive aspects of her sovereignty transcend the boundaries of her personal sphere, and rest on how this personal sphere is connected and related to others.

Consider now what this could mean for *data* sovereignty. In the case of data sovereignty, the relevant kind of power is control over one's data: where it goes, who has access, and what is being done with it. The foregoing suggests that the individual need not always exercise sovereignty in ways that close off her personal data from others, e.g., by categorically prioritizing her right to privacy. As proponents of relational autonomy highlight, persons are not just independent, isolated, and self-interested beings (Mackenzie and Stoljar 2000; Dabrock et al. 2004; Baylis et al. 2008; Dabrock 2012; Steinfath and Wiesemann 2016; Braun 2017). Their selfhood and well-being depend on rich and complex relations to others, their community, and society as a whole. Importantly, this can mean that the data sovereign individual does not just close off her data, but *shares* it with others. In fact, practices of sharing one's personal data can constitute meaningful advances and reinforcements of the social structures in which the individual seeks to realize positive aspects of her sovereignty (see also Barbara Prainsack's contribution to this volume for a discussion of the relational nature of donations). This is a particularly fruitful option if these acts of sharing take the form of donating and endowing.

In his seminal discussion, Mauss (1950) describes a range of features which he claims are distinctive of the notion of a gift. When someone gives goods in the context of a trade, she expects a return. In contrast, while a gift might be tied to reciprocal obligations between donor and recipient, it always points to something beyond these. A gift is tied to the donor's generosity as well as some form of obligation on the side of the recipient. In this sense, there is a similarity with economic exchange because the relationship that is being constituted through the act of giving is two-ways, mutual, or symmetrical. Still, the character of the gift cannot be captured in terms of the logic of exchange: the reciprocal obligations in question are incommensurable and cannot be set off against each other in an economic calculus. Gifts might not be incompatible with trade and exchange, but they involve much more. They provide systematic means for individuals and groups to articulate and reciprocate recognition, and thereby determine and shape identities. "[B]y giving one is giving *oneself*, and if one gives oneself, it is because one 'owes' *oneself*—one's person and one's goods—to others" (Mauss 1950, p. 59).

Other authors insist that gifts need to be distinguished more sharply from exchange. For example, Derrida argues that a genuine gift cannot involve expectations of reciprocation of any kind. The gift "interrupts economy", "suspends economic calculation", "def[ies] reciprocity or symmetry", remains outside the "circle" of economic exchange, and is thus distinctively "*aneconomic*" (Derrida 1992, p. 7). One important consequence is that once the recipient perceives and recognizes the gift as a gift, it is "annulled" or "destroyed" as the act of giving becomes situated within a logic of exchange. Mere recognition of the gift as a gift already "gives back" (Derrida 1992, p. 13). In fact, not even the donor may be aware of the gift; otherwise the donor threatens "to pay himself with a symbolic recognition, to praise himself, to approve of himself, to gratify himself, to congratulate himself, to give back to himself symbolically" (Derrida 1992, p. 14). Because awareness and recognition annul the gift, the notion is inherently aporetic, and genuine gifts are impossible. Nevertheless, Derrida argues that it is out of the question to refrain from giving. He suggests that the gift is actually fundamental to exchange; giving is what "puts the economy in motion". We need to

> "engage in the effort of thinking or rethinking a sort of transcendental illusion of the gift. [...] *Know* still what giving *wants to say, know how to give*, know what you want and want to say when you give, know what you intend to give, know how the gift annuls itself, commit yourself [*engage-toi*] even if commitment is the destruction of the gift by the gift, give economy its chance" (Derrida 1992, p. 30; his italics).

Hénaff too insists that the gift has certain unique features. He distinguishes *symbolic* from *economic* exchange. Drawing on Mauss, he agrees that gifts figure in *symbolic* exchanges whose purpose is to establish and foster social bonds through relations of recognition, honour, and esteem amongst parties. It also prompts and articulates attitudes of generosity, benevolence, and gratefulness. Such *symbolic* exchange is "entirely outside the circuit of what is useful and profitable" (Hénaff 2010, p. 18). He criticizes that Mauss' discussion is not always consistent about the non-economic and non-commodifiable aspects of the gift as *symbolic* exchange (Hénaff 2010, p. 110). Hénaff further provides a threefold typology of the gift: *ceremonial* gifts which are public and reciprocal, *gracious* ones which are private and unilateral, and *mutual aid* which pertains to solidaric or philanthropic activity

(Hénaff 2013, pp. 15–6). The mutual and public character of the ceremonial gift ties it to practices of recognition and attributions of equality in public space; it accounts for its central role in "*identifying*, *accepting*, and finally *honoring* others" (Hénaff 2013, p. 19; his italics). He proposes that these characteristic features of ceremonial token gifts ultimately culminate in political and legal institutions that protect and guarantee recognition (Hénaff 2013, pp. 21–2) and, amongst others, open up room for gracious gifts and mutual aid.

Ricœur is convinced that appreciating a gift need not take the form of a restitution that annuls it. What matters is the way in which the gift is received. If the gift succeeds in bringing about a kind of gratefulness that acknowledges the donor's generosity *without* forcing or pressuring the recipient to reciprocate, then appearances of aporia and impossibility can be circumvented. "Gratitude lightens the weight of obligation to give in return and reorients this toward a generosity equal to the one that led to the first gift" (Ricœur 2005, p. 244). One important consequence is that *ex ante*, it must remain open whether this orientation towards the donor's generosity actually occurs. If the recipient reciprocates, she does so freely and without duty. A genuine gift involves openness and contingency. It cannot be forced or guided.

As Mauss and Hénaff highlight, the gift can function as a source and catalyst for recognition. It does so by reflecting an endowment of the donor, a symbolic dimension through which the donor dedicates her gift and conveys a meaning beyond the commodifiable aspects of the good being given. In Mauss' view, the donor blends *herself* with the good being given. "Souls are mixed with things; things with souls. Lives are mingled together, and this is how, among persons and things so intermingled, each emerges from their own sphere and mixes together" (Mauss 1950, pp. 25–6). If through dedications of this kind, the donor manages to establish social bonds or even—in Derrida's words—to *interrupt* patterns of economic exchange, then the gift extends the individual's room for manoeuvre in social space. It opens up options for shaping and enhancing interactions and deepening modes of integration among individuals.

The mentioned authors disagree whether gifts should be understood as being diametrally opposed to economic exchange, or whether they, too, can involve mutual expectations, obligations, and relations of reciprocity. The latter seems plausible in view of the fact that through making a gift, the donor exposes herself to others and thereby engages in a potentially precarious gamble (Braun 2017, pp. 206–7). With regards to potlach ceremonies, Mauss notes that "to lose one's prestige is to lose one's soul. It is in fact the 'face', the dancing mask, the right to incarnate a spirit, to wear a coat of arms, a totem, it is really the *persona*—that are all called into question in this way, and that are lost at the potlach, at the game of gifts, just as they can be lost in war, or through a mistake in ritual" (Mauss 1950, p. 50). Gifts are attempts at giving and seeking recognition. Such attempts can fail in various ways. They can be confirmed and reciprocated, but also disappoint, overburden, be perceived as coercive, or simply not be met with gratefulness. Thus, there is no need to romanticize gifts. They can open up opportunities, but they can also generate burdens or injustices. Moreover, the donor can face reactions and structures that reject her attempts to give. By making, enabling, or accepting gifts, we have not established fairness, not even ruled out violence. Gifts can only set the stage for negotiating these aspects.

In the acts of giving discussed by Mauss, Derrida, Hénaff, Ricœur and others, two dimensions can be distinguished: first, there is an aspect of *exchange* insofar as these acts of giving involve transfers of goods and expectations of some form of return or reciprocation, assessed against the backdrop of an economic rationale or logic. Second, there is a distinctive *gift* aspect which expresses recognition and valuation of the recipient and thus yields community-sustaining potentials. The appropriateness and success of such expressive acts is assessed relative to a logic of recognition. For the sake of speaking in a theory-neutral fashion and not beg any questions against authors like Derrida who think the former aspect actually undermines the latter, we suggest the term 'donation' as denoting acts of giving for which it is conceptually open whether they encompass exchange and/or gift aspects. Considering only one of those dimensions would fall short of capturing the complexity of the target phenomenon. In the resulting picture, donations need not be entirely distinct from exchange, yet they are something over and above it. In the words of Waldenfels (2012), donations *exceed* relations of mere exchange.

Practices of organ and blood donation impact recipients in an immediate, intimate, and bodily way and are sometimes characterized as instantiating central features highlighted by Mauss' analysis: the presence and reinforcement of institutions that enable donations, expectations and even subtle pressures that motivate individuals to give, obligations on the side of the recipient to accept the gift, and recipients who are expected *and* feel the need to reciprocate (Fox and Swazey 1978; Vernale and Packard 1990; Sque and Payne 1994; Gill and Lowes 2008). In line with the insight that donations are risky and their effects contingent, organ and blood donations can impose undue burdens on recipients and effectively establish a "tyranny of the gift" (Fox and Swazey 1978, p. 383). Gift-theoretic insights on the entanglement between giving, gratuity, and gratification further resonate with recent work inspired by the conceptions of relational autonomy just mentioned. One of the consequences of the complex interplay between selfhood and orientation towards others is that motivations for acts of giving often cannot be straightforwardly classified as either altruistic or self-interested. Apparently altruistic donations carry aspects of self-interest and vice versa. In particular, empirical work suggests a "simultaneity of self-interested and other-regarding practice in the field of organ donation "(Prainsack 2018; cf. also Simpson 2018).

Technological innovations and their impact on research and clinical care prompt us to focus on the provision of personal health data as a new and promising way to affect others. We shall discuss some opportunities below (3.). Importantly, most people who make health-related donations do not give in these ways in order to generate a return. This suggests that a logic of exchange cannot fully explain what is happening, and the gift paradigm might be able to go some way towards explaining core features of these practices.

If we buy into the idea that sovereignty means more than the right and power to keep others from interfering with one's personal sphere and is realized at least in part along outward-reaching, interactive and participatory dimensions, then donations could advance these positive aspects of sovereignty. Donations are surely just one amongst many ways to enter into relations with others, but their *aneconomic* aspects promise some distinctive community- and recognition-sustaining opportunities. Insofar as data sovereignty, and especially its positive dimension, is a worthwhile normative target notion, individuals should be enabled to donate personal health data. As we will argue, this is compatible with insisting on a range of mechanisms and safeguards to ensure that tensions between positive sovereignty and the protective aspects of its negative counterpart are minimized.

3.3 Reasons in Favour of Data Donations

In the following, we highlight three ways in which data donations could advance positive data sovereignty.

3.3.1 Solidarity

Data donations can express solidarity. Although not used uniformly throughout the literature, Prainsack and Buyx propose that the concept of solidarity involves "shared practices reflecting a collective commitment to carry 'costs' (financial, social, emotional, or otherwise) to assist others" (2012, p. 346; italics removed). Data donations fall under this definition insofar as they reflect the willingness to share efforts that are essential for advancing research and thereby helping those who are in need of findings and innovations. Prainsack and Buyx add the further condition that this willingness is based on the donor "recogniz[ing] sameness or similarity in at least one relevant respect" (2012, p. 346; italics removed)—a condition that distinguishes solidarity from altruism and charity, which do not necessarily rest on an understanding of symmetry between the agent and the recipient. Data donations meet this recognition-of-similarity constraint, too. This is obvious if—as on PatientsLikeMe—the donor is providing her data for the benefit of individuals who share her risk profile or illness. But even if motivations differ and/or it is not clear who exactly will benefit from the data, we can suppose that the donor's contribution is at least partly based on the insight that she herself could one day find herself in a situation where she benefits from donations of this kind, and so recognizes similarity with the beneficiary in a relevant respect.

Two examples illustrate how the gathering and sharing of data can relate to solidarity. First, generating data about oneself, whether through genetic testing or by means of self-tracking devices like wearables and other new technologies, might appear egoistic, solipsistic, or self-centred. However, it can have an inherently social and communicative dimension (cf. Sharon 2017, pp. 111–2; Ajana 2018, p. 128). Such data gathering is being carried out not only to further one's own ends, but also to share, report, discuss, and compare one's data with others.

Second, consider the importance of data gatherers and contributors for personalized medicine. Personalization of health services might appear individualistic insofar as it focuses on specific traits of a given patient, and increasingly shifts responsibility for health towards the individual. But alternatively, personalized medicine can be seen as a context in which individual and collective good are inherently intertwined. Individual health tracking, testing, and data-sharing are key towards building up the databases that enable tailor-made health services. Through this "bottom-up" process from self-tracking to the generation of common knowledge bases, there is a sense in which personalization of services rests on "the idea that the overall health [...] of the population can only be improved if individuals take on more personal responsibility for their own health"; we arrive at an "intertwining of the personal and collective good" (Sharon 2017, p. 100).

3.3.2 *Beneficence*

Donating data promises "New Opportunities to Enrich Understanding of Individual and Population Health" (Health Data Exploration Project 2014). Research attains public goods such as knowledge, technology, and health. Data is one essential ingredient in research success. In the age of wearables, smartphones, and other self-tracking devices, plenty of personal health data is being generated. However, most of it remains inaccessible to medical and public health research. Data donations could allow the research community to utilize generated data and to convert it into predictions, treatments, and other innovations that potentially benefit a great number of patients, health systems, and populations. In the ideal case, these benefits come at minimal costs for the donors. Unlike organ donation, data donation doesn't hurt. It is convenient and effortless. And unlike donations to charities, there is no financial burden for the donor.

Data donations can also lead to self-interested benefits. The PatientsLikeMe campaign claims that donating one's data also helps "to improve one's own condition" (2014), and DNA.land (2018) promises to reveal new insights about the donor's genome. At the very least, contributing to a common practice of data donations adds to improved evidence bases, understanding of diseases, and treatments that ameliorate clinical practice. It is also possible that the provision and analysis of data leads to the discovery of actionable incidental findings that would have otherwise remained unnoticed. Only upon receiving this information can the donor take preventive and curative steps.

There are many potential beneficiaries of data donations. Data helps foundational science, doctors, patients, healthy individuals, society as a whole, insurers, and others (German Ethics Council 2017a, sect. 4.4). Moreover, there is a plurality of services that can be ameliorated: knowledge generation and supply, diagnosis, prediction, treatment. Improvements can be achieved along several dimensions: in terms of the hedonic benefits they provide, the costs they save, and/or the contributions they make to social integration.

3.3.3 Participation

The significance and normative dimension of scientific research need not be exhausted by the benefits it generates. Focusing on genomic research, Knoppers et al. argue that a human right to benefit from science includes the right "to have access to and share in both the development and fruits of science across the translation continuum, from basic research through practical, material application" (2014, p. 899). In a similar vein, Vayena and Tasioulas (2015, 2016) argue that science is a central component of the kind of communal and cultural life to which all humans are entitled. The authors highlight an underappreciated *participatory* dimension of the right to science: human rights frameworks like the Universal Declaration of Human Rights (1948, art. 27) and the International Covenant on Economic, Social and Cultural Rights (1966, art. 15) entitle individuals to *take part in* scientific endeavours. Encouraging and enabling data donations would certainly be an important step towards respecting this right and including broader populations in scientific endeavours. Proponents of a participatory right to science could even insist that mere data gathering and sharing falls short of respecting the right to science in all its facets. Understood more comprehensively, it also entitles individuals to participation in financing, agenda setting, governance, and even lead roles in initiating, designing, and carrying out studies. The human right to science imposes duties

> "to equip people with the basic scientific knowledge needed to participate in science or to provide citizen scientists with various forms of support and recognition, e.g. sources of research funding, access to oversight mechanisms and the opportunity to publish in scientific journals" (Vayena and Tasioulas 2015, p. 482).

According to such positions, strong reasons in favour of enabling data donations actually imply that we shouldn't stop there, but enable much more.

3.4 Challenges with Data Donations

Data donations can provide great benefits, express and foster solidarity, and enable individuals to participate in scientific research. But they also raise some difficulties and puzzles.

3.4.1 Trust

One aspect that well-established practices of giving like financial, organ, or blood donations share with data donations is their reliance on trust. They function only if the donor can expect that her willingness to give will not be exploited by collectors and facilitators, that her donation is being handled responsibly and put to work effectively, and that no third-party interests interfere with the equitable distribution of her donation. The donor also expects that her contributions are being made against the backdrop of appropriate safeguards that protect her from harm, and that burdens arising from the donation process are minimized. Important questions arise about which institutional designs best promote that such expectations are met, trust does not erode, and the practice remains stable. Data donations presuppose trust in similar ways. One case in point is the backlash against the NHS care.data scheme in the United Kingdom, which was intended to enable the sharing of personal health data for research, but was met with distrust due to shortcomings in communication and transparency (Sterckx et al. 2016).

3.4.2 Future Use

The scope and timing of financial, organ, or blood donations is clearly defined. Donations of biological specimen can be sought with a reasonably well-defined purpose in mind, but already here questions loom about admissible future uses of such samples beyond the initially intended purpose. For example, after plenty of samples were collected to speed up research and development efforts during the 2014 outbreak of the Ebola virus disease in West Africa, question arose about how to use these biobanks responsibly in a way that provides long-term benefits for the health systems and scientific infrastructures of affected countries (Hayden 2015; World Health Organization 2015). Unlike organ and blood donations, biological specimen are not exhausted once they reach a beneficiary. They can be analysed repeatedly in a variety of study designs. To harness these potentials, regulators and researchers need to think carefully about consent mechanisms, the provision of appropriate information to sample donors, and mechanisms to govern access to the biobanks in which samples are stored.

One distinctive feature of data donations is that the possibility of future uses familiar from biobank donations is driven to the extreme. Consider the de- and recontextualization processes which datasets tend to undergo in the age of big data. Donated health data is likely to be processed and analysed by means of algorithms and applications that are designed to discover and examine unforeseen correlation hypotheses (cf. Mittelstadt and Floridi 2016, p. 312). From a normative perspective, this raises at least three issues.

First, the protective value of anonymization is limited. Some data, such as genomic information, is essentially personalized and cannot be anonymized. But even for other kinds of information, the possibility of de- and recontextualization entails that deanonymization cannot be ruled out. Giving data might be relatively convenient and effortless, but depending on the kind of data and context, such linkages can have quite significant consequences. Surprising inferences can be drawn from personal information especially once it is combined with and set in relation to other data sets. The problem is that individuals are less and less in a position to foresee and take into account potential harms and/or disadvantages that can accrue on the individual or the collective level.

Second, because future uses and possible inferences about the data subject are to some extent unclear at the point of data collection, it is challenging to design consent mechanisms that *inform* individuals appropriately. The problem is not just that non-experts lack the competence to foresee the possibilities of recontextualization and linkage with other data sets, and that this leads to deep asymmetries of information between data donor and users who have the expertise and technology to process it. At the point of donation, the range of possible recontextualizations, linkages, and inferences can remain inaccessible even to experts. In other words, the exact quality and character of the donation is in constant flux. The question arises how under these conditions, an individual can meaningfully deliberate upon whether or not to donate her health data. There is a tension between the very idea of making such a donation, and the fact that it must remain somewhat opaque to both donors and collectors what exactly is being donated.

Third, the availability of greater sets of data by itself does not guarantee improvements in the quality of data and/or the inferences drawn from it. The complexity of big data sets and the tools used to analyse them poses a range of epistemic challenges for data collectors and researchers that complicate the evaluation of big-data-driven hypotheses (cf. Mittelstadt and Floridi 2016, p. 327). The beneficent potential of data donations is directly tied to the scientific soundness of their analysis, processing, and conversion into research and development. Providing her data entitles the donor to reasonable expectations towards the scientific institutions whom she authorizes to use and leverage her donation, for example the expectation that her data is being used responsibly and effectively in a way that reflects her philanthropic intentions. These expectations will get frustrated if scientific virtues like rigour, care, and modesty are not enacted consistently throughout data collection, analysis, and interpretation.

3.4.3 Invasiveness

The implications about asymmetries of information become even more significant once we consider how invasive data can be in the age of big data, genomics, and continuous and holistic tracking. When we speak of data that can be donated, we are referring to a vast number of biological markers such as an individual's complete and unique set of genetic information, physical parameters such as location and movements, lifestyle data, and even data about emotions, moods, and states of mind. Moreover, linkages amongst datasets lead to *cumulative effects* (Braun and Dabrock 2016a, pp. 316–7). First, the combination of clinical records with data from medical research, self-tracking technologies like fitness apps, lifestyle data, financial data, etc. results in levels of invasiveness which individual datasets do not achieve. Second, distinctions between seemingly discrete data kinds and spheres begin to vanish. The fact that companies like Apple, Google, and Microsoft are already active in all these domains underlines that linkages between them are only a matter of time.

The penetrative character of data and devices means that what they extract from us transcends concepts like parthood or possession. The German philosopher Helmuth Plessner (1980) has drawn a distinction between physical body (*Körper*) and living body (*Leib*). According to Plessner, one distinctive feature of human life is eccentric positionality, i.e. a particular mode of relating to its own positionality in space: humans can conceive of themselves as both physical bodies existing in the corporeal, outer world of things *and* as experiencing selves occupying the centre of a spatially delineated physical body, the locus of perceptions, actions, and experiences (cf. also de Mul 2014). Qua physical body, humans *live*, but qua living bodies, humans are subjects of *experienced life*. This double aspect is reflected by the two simultaneously instantiated modes of *being* a living body (*Leibsein*) and *having* a physical body (*Körperhaben*). In view of these concepts and distinctions introduced by Plessner, we might wonder whether, once individuals and their experiences are seen as complex conglomerates of algorithmic processes (for example Harari 2016 chs. 2, 10, 11), captured in their entirety by holistic, rich datasets and invasive devices, the difference between what we *are* and the features we *have* has collapsed. In this case, some kinds of data donations—the ones paradigmatically enabled by novel big data technologies—would involve much more than donating merely a *part* of me, or merely something *about* me. The question arises what about me is *not* being captured by data. As long as it remains unanswered, we are left with a sense in which the data donor can give *all of her, all she is*. The scope of the potential donation is unprecedented.

3.4.4 Ownership

In order to donate something, it must be mine. I cannot donate things that belong to you, such as your blood or organs. My personal health data is certainly about me, but is it also mine? Much seems to depend on the sense of ownership in question. For example, it is contentious whether personal health data can be seen as private property. Montgomery offers several reasons to reject the suggestion. He notes that in the context of health data, intuitions about privacy "sit uneasily with property ideas": even if we commodify personal health data, "information 'about me' does not cease to be connected to my privacy when I give (or sell) it to others" (Montgomery 2017, p. 82). This suggests that ownership in the sense of private property is not primarily what motivates the regulation of health data.

Moreover, according to a broadly Lockean account, private property results from mixing labour with resources. This idea undercuts rather than supports the view that my health data is mine. While I might have "invest[ed] bodily samples" (Montgomery 2017, p. 83), it is the medical service provider who analyses specimen and data, compiles it into evidence bases, and generates value based on the raw materials I am providing. If labour is any indication, then "[i]f anyone may claim proprietary rights over the information on the labour theory of property, it would seem to be the health professionals or service for which they work" (Montgomery 2017, p. 84).

Montgomery suggests that if we really want to regard data like genomic information as property, it should not be considered *private*. One alternative is to regard such data *as common* property, i.e. property shared by a group of people (such as families) and outsiders being excluded. But Montgomery himself prefers the paradigm of *public* property: genomic data is like the air we breathe in the sense that everybody is entitled to it, the resource is not exhausted by universal access, and the benefits connected to its usage motivate obligations of stewardship and preservation.

We might have to complement such an account with the additional thesis that privacy- rather than property-related claims could still exclude access to personal health data, especially given the degree of invasiveness and comprehensiveness described above. What matters for our purposes is that data donations are disanalogous to other ways of giving in that they do not involve a transfer of something the donor owns in a straightforward way (on this issue, see also Barbara Prainsack's contribution to this volume). In fact, as Montgomery also notes, data donations need not even involve a *transfer*: the data donor need not *lose* anything. Instead, her donation might be best understood as a suspension of certain privacy claims.

Considerations about ownership become highly relevant once calls for data donations are addressed not only at individuals, but also at data-processing organizations and institutions. In this context, *data philanthropy* refers to the provision of data from private sector silos for the public benefit, e.g., development aid, disaster relief efforts, and public health surveillance. Social media data can be key in the detection and monitoring of disease outbreaks. Organizations could share data of this kind not only on the basis of corporate social responsibility, but because they recognize the need for a "real-time data commons" (Kirkpatrick 2013). One necessary condition is that the privacy of individuals can be protected through measures like anonymization and aggregation. Even in cases where this is not possible, the hope is that "more sensitive data [...] is nevertheless analysed by companies behind their firewalls for specific smoke signals" (Kirkpatrick 2011). Since such data is generated by the private entity, typically on the basis of some form of consent, there is a sense in which this entity is the *owner*. However, the owner and envisioned data philanthropist is not the *data subject*. It must be ensured that the interests of the latter are not compromised when data is being made available.

3.4.5 Affected People

In organ or blood donations, the identity of the beneficiary is often somewhat unclear: unless I am donating to a relative or friend, the recipient will be some indeterminate or unfamiliar other who is in need of the materials I am providing. Still, I have at least a vague idea about certain features and needs of the recipient, e.g., that she is in need of an organ. Something similar applies if I disclose personal health data for the benefit of people who share my illness or risk profile, e.g., on PatientsLikeMe. But note that once data is either decontextualized as described above or not being donated with such a specific purpose in mind, e.g., when uploading one's genome on openSNP, the potential beneficiary and the way in which she benefits from the contribution become increasingly abstract.

Not only does the range of beneficiaries of the data donation broaden—it is also less clear who is carrying the burdens and consequences connected with the act of sharing. The donation of my kidney is a sacrifice which I make myself. Setting aside the beneficiary, the effects of my donation on others are minimal. In particular, any burdens related to the donation are carried almost exclusively by myself. In contrast, consider how submitting my genome to a public database could reveal information not only about myself, but also about my children or relatives, e.g., on hereditary risk factors. The range of people being affected as well as the precise consequences of the donation are much less transparent to the donor than in other health-related donations.

3.4.6 Voluntariness

Donations are conscious, deliberate, uncoerced acts of giving, informed by beliefs about a need that is being addressed through the donation. Data donations can be made by means explicit provision of information towards research projects and platforms, or by accepting terms and conditions of platforms that gather, evaluate, and maybe even publish data of its users (Kostkova et al. 2016). In any case, the informed will of the donor cannot be bypassed. In this context, at least two challenges arise.

First, there is a risk of opacity or even deception about the purpose of data gathering, especially if the sharing of data offers significant benefits to private sector service providers. The question arises how societies and individual donors choose to evaluate the activities of commercial entities who convert philanthropic data donations into products that might improve lives to some extent, but in the first place generate non-altruistic, self-serving revenues. For example, the biotechnology company 23andMe (2018) motivates customers to become "part of something bigger" and make contributions that "help drive scientific discoveries" by allowing the company to use data from its direct-to-consumer genetic testing services for research purposes. At the same time, 23andMe is generating intellectual property from its biobank, such as the patent of a gene sequence which it found to contribute to the risk of developing Alzheimer disease (Hayden 2012), and a method for gamete donor selection that allows prospective parents to select for desired traits in their future child (Sterckx et al. 2013).

Calls for data donations may allude to philanthropy, altruism, solidarity, and the good a donation can do, but in fact they might at least partly be driven by the self-interest of the data collector. The question of whether to share data in view of private sector benefits becomes particularly pressing in contexts where the latter *conflict* with the donor's beneficent aims. For example, consider a situation in which data provision that is intended as philanthropic advances medical research while enhancing and stratifying insurers' knowledge about risk profiles of donors and customers.

Such prospects can ultimately deter individuals from sharing. If not, it provides opportunities for private sector entities to freeride upon philanthropic dispositions.

Second, the informed will of the potential donor can be challenged by apparent moral pressures. Understood charitably, headlines like "Our Health Data Can Save Lives, But We Have to Be Willing to Share" (Gent 2017) can be seen as raising awareness for so far unrecognized, readily available, and effort-efficient means for the individual to improve the lives of others. But there is a somewhat questionable flipside to such statements. They might be taken to suggest that an individual acts wrongly if she ultimately prioritizes her privacy over the presumed benefits of a data donation, and/or if she judges the privacy risks to be disproportionate relative to the utility that would be generated by her donation. In other words, a perceived duty to participate might result (Bialobrzeski et al. 2012). In view of rhetoric that declares data a common good and public asset, Ajana sees a risk of pitting data philanthropists against privacy advocates when

> "in the name of altruism and public good, individuals and organisations are subtly being encouraged to prioritise sharing and contributing over maintaining privacy. [...] First, it reinforces [...] the misleading assumption that individuals wishing to keep their data private are either selfish and desire privacy because they are not interested in helping others, or bad and desire privacy to hide negative acts and information. Second, this binary thinking also underlies the misconception that privacy is a purely individual right and does not extend to society at large" (Ajana 2018, pp. 133–4).

A parallel can be drawn to worries regarding self-imposed surveillance and disciplining mechanisms (Foucault 1977) through self-tracking devices (Sharon 2017, pp. 98–99). Voluntary tracking and provision of personal health data can turn into liberty-constraining expectations that data is not only shared, but also that individuals take measures to improve their health markers (Braun and Dabrock 2016a, p. 323). The prospect of doing good with one's data can similarly be turned into a disciplining narrative that conveys implicit expectations that data should not be withheld. What initially appears to open up options for the individual ends up delimiting them.

These dynamics would be unfortunate from a normative perspective. Data donations might be beneficial and morally commendable, and these features provide *some* reason to donate. But they hardly provide an all-things-considered reason—let alone a strict duty—to do so. Consider two examples: first, for the Kantian, the duty to help others is an imperfect one, i.e. it remains entirely up to the agent to what extent she helps others (Kant 1785, p. 423). Second, consider *effective altruism* according to which there are strong moral reasons to give, e.g., donating money to charity, organs to patients in need, or time and labour to good causes (Singer 2009, 2015; MacAskill 2015), but also to ensure that the good your efforts bring about is being maximized. To our knowledge, *effective altruists* have not yet explored data donations, but they could be intrigued by the benefits that can be realized through such acts of giving. Still, *effective altruists* agree that although *once* you donate, you should donate as effectively as possible, there can be *optionality* about *whether* to donate at all. Strong normative reasons to give money to charity can be *outweighed* by the costs such donations incur to the donor. In such cases, "it would not be wrong of you to do nothing" (Pummer 2016, p. 81). According to these positions, it is far from unreasonable or immoral if an individual decides to be restrictive about her data. It is a fine line between holding her contributions in esteem and implicitly sanctioning or generating a burden of proof for the individual who decides to keep her information restricted.

To sum up, donating personal health data offers alluring opportunities (3.), but a number of challenges lurk along the way. Genuine donors typically have some idea about what they are donating, what the donation will be used for, whom it benefits, and who carries burdens related to the donation. However, in big data contexts, potential data donors are bound to have a limited grip on the nature of their donation, the future use of their data, and the people affected by their decision to share. Further disanalogies come from the invasive and comprehensive character of state-of-the-art data gathering and processing, and the fact that the relevant sense of ownership is far from straightforward. Finally, the voluntariness of data donations can be undercut by opaque or deceptive information and/or moral pressures that appear to deflate individual privacy claims.

Earlier, we suggested that donations can advance positive data sovereignty as they foster social bonds and open up room for manoeuvre in social space. Specifically, we suggested that through data donations, individuals can enact beneficence, solidarity, and play an active role in scientific processes. The challenges just characterized aggravate the uncertainties that are inherent to any act of giving. Important aspects of the good being given are in constant flux—what it will be used for, whom it benefits, and who carries burdens. If the donor decides to give nevertheless, she embarks on a venture into the unknown that can become precarious. Not only might the donation be in vain, fail to accord with the donor's intentions, and remain unsuccessful in advancing positive sovereignty. Even worse, the donation could backfire and end up compromising negative aspects of the donor's sovereignty that relate to protective claims and rights, for example against untoward interferences from others, disadvantages, discrimination, or exploitation.

3.5 Donations, Consent and Control

As mentioned earlier (2.), one important realizer of sovereignty is power. In the case of data sovereignty, the relevant power is control over one's data. The question arises how data donations can be facilitated and regulated in a way that guards and strengthens the data sovereignty of potential donors. We now suggest three governance areas that are crucial towards this goal. Ideally, mechanisms in these areas enable potential donors to contribute their health data for the benefit of others and scientific progress as a whole without leaving them susceptible to undue harms arising from the aforementioned challenges.

3.5.1 Consent

Several initiatives highlight a considerable degree of willingness on the side of individuals to share their data (Wellcome Trust 2013; Health Data Exploration Project 2014; PatientsLikeMe 2014). However, it has also been recognized the willingness to share data, and especially preferences about what kind of data may be shared, is expected to vary amongst user groups (Weitzman et al. 2010). The example of the care.data scheme shows that sharing and connecting health data can prompt scepticism as soon as insufficient attention is being devoted to the consent of data subjects. It is thus necessary to focus on the conditions and mechanisms for meaningful, informed decision-making. As mentioned, many uncertainties surround the future use of one's data. In big data contexts, the informedness of one-time consent to data gathering and processing inevitably remains incomplete (Mittelstadt and Floridi 2016, p. 312). Given the prospective benefits of data donations outlined earlier, and the potentials of big data methods more generally, it stands to reason to not simply refrain from useful activities in the absence of fully informed consent, but to rethink and redesign informed consent in a way that makes these activities possible *and* honours the data subject's self-determination. Even if data is already collected and in principle available for analysis, it is highly questionable whether informed consent can legitimately be bypassed (Ioannidis 2013). And needless to say, for our context it matters that data crawling and processing without consent undermines the very idea of a data *donation*.

A range of new consent forms are under discussion in the literature. Reliance on opt-out mechanisms in biobanks and online data gathering (CIOMS 2016, chs. 11, 22) is already widespread. Blanket consent poses little to no constraints on future uses. Broad consent allows a wide range of future uses (Petrini 2010). Tiered consent can take several forms, from the specification of a range of approved uses, to the exclusion of certain uses, to requiring re-consent if usage for a new purpose is intended (Eiseman et al. 2003, pp. 134–7; Master et al. 2015).

Each of these options can enable valuable research, but also compromises the ideal of informed consent to some extent. For example, they do not satisfy the standards of informedness laid out in the Declaration of Helsinki (World Medical Association 1964). Some thus argue, e.g., that "blanket consents cannot be considered true consent" (Caulfield et al. 2003) since it is provided on the basis of information that is way too vague and does not allow the individual to act on her continuing interest in her health information. Others even conclude that *informed* consent is inapplicable to contexts like biobanking where uncertainty about future use is unavoidable (Cargill 2016).

In fact, we must highlight a further problem. Inherent to alternative consent models is typically a more or less explicit distinction between *sectors*. Information and samples are being given for a certain range of future uses or certain tiers of research. Oversight mechanisms and committees are thus needed to determine whether a particular usage request of a researcher accords with the consent provided at enrolment. But note how given our earlier remarks about future use and de- and recontextualization, these sectorial distinctions are in jeopardy in big data contexts. For example, consider the consent to the processing of one's social media data, given through acceptance of terms and conditions (Kostkova et al. 2016, p. 2). Once analysed by suitable algorithms and linked with other data sets, certain social media data (or metadata) effectively becomes health data. Of course, this can be seen as a challenge already for single-instance consent, given that it becomes increasingly less transparent to the individual what can and will be done with her data. But novel consent forms become even more tricky once the sectorial distinctions inherent to broad or tiered consent forms fade.

Problems like these motivate consent forms that are *dynamic*. Different individuals possess different preferences depending on the kind and context of data in question. Moreover, preferences can be expected to change over time, for example if technological advances open up new possibilities for drawing inferences from a given dataset. This calls for *refined* and *dynamic* control mechanisms that allow individuals to provide and withdraw data in accordance with their evolving preferences—a demand which has found its way into legislation on data portability, e.g., in Article 20 of the EU General Data Protection Regulation (GDPR). Once individuals become equipped with effective means to access and transfer their data, they turn from mere data subjects to active data *distributors* (Vayena and Blasimme 2017, pp. 507–8).

One example for what this could mean for data donations is provided by Schapranow et al. (2017). While organ donation passes are common, similar mechanisms are lacking for data donations. The authors thus introduce a *data donation pass*, which can be maintained through a smartphone app in which individuals can choose in real-time whether and for how long they would like to provide their data to research projects, what kind of projects they would like to support, what kind of data is being shared, and when it shall be withdrawn. Besides highlighting potential benefits, the authors explicitly construe the data donation pass as a means for the individual to exercise data sovereignty.

3.5.2 Representation

Innovative consent forms can be complemented by representatives who express or represent the donor's will in governance processes. For example, trustee or honest broker models authorize a neutral and unbiased individual, committee, or system to manage access requests by researchers and function as a firewall between the database and potential data processors (Vaught and Lockhart 2012). The purpose of honest brokers is typically to secure the privacy and anonymity of individuals. We can easily imagine extending its scope to representing further interests of the donor. In this context, we might also invoke the concept of *custodianship*, which aims at ensuring accountability to the data donor across the full spectrum from data collection to database maintenance and access permission.

> "Custodianship does not entail the right to ownership but acknowledges that a biospecimen is provided to research as a 'gift' to be used only with consent to advance science for the benefit of society" (Yassin et al. 2010).

Going one step further, one can take on board some of the ideas from *citizen science* indicated earlier. For example, Shirk et al. (2012) distinguish several models of public involvement in scientific research. Such models could also be applied when including data subjects in governance processes: on one end of the spectrum, individuals are merely *contributing* data or specimen to research projects. In *collaborative* projects, donors or members of the refine research project designs together with investigators. In *co-created* projects, researchers and donors work as equals. And in *collegial* contributions, non-credentialed individuals even carry out research independently.

3.5.3 Organizations

Data sovereignty appears as a feature of individuals, but consent structures, participatory designs, and organizational self-control set the stage for it. Shaping these structures in a way conducive to data sovereignty is indispensable. This requires organization-level commitments and rules prompted by a thoughtful mix of incentives and frameworks along at least two dimensions. First, mechanisms of voluntary self-control, either on the level of corporate social responsibility, or by setting up industry-wide, impartial licensing and control agencies should be considered. Second, the state can intervene by reshaping legislation for the operation of data-processing institutions, e.g., through the mentioned EU GDPR. Either way, data sharing requirements need to be designed with care. For example, there is a potential tension between *mandatory publication* of publicly funded data and the willingness of individuals to donate. The former can speed up research, but also—especially in the case of genomic data—increase privacy risks and thus deter potential donors.

3.5.4 Observation I

In the literature, it is sometimes noted that data donations solve problems with research in which standard informed consent is impracticable. The idea is that in view of looming deanonymization, de- and recontextualization, and future uses, research is bound to rely on "information altruists" (Kohane and Altman 2005) who are aware of these risks, but share their data nevertheless. On the far end of the spectrum is probably the OpenSNP case where whole genomes are freely accessible. The upshot is that people who are willing to take risks facilitate research that would otherwise be impossible or very hard to carry out, while the consent requirements for the general, less risk-seeking public remain uncompromised.

We saw earlier that sovereignty can indeed be transferred and delegated to others. But we also saw that considerations about the legitimacy of the sovereign indicate that obligations of representation and accountability are tied to such transfers. Sovereigns who fail to represent their people are despots. Moreover, on reflection we might become convinced that certain fundamental aspects of individual sovereignty resist transfer to others. As Judith Butler puts it, when people vote, "[s]omething of popular sovereignty remains untranslatable, non-transferable, and even unsubstitutable, which is why it can both elect and dissolve regimes" (2015, p. 162). The implication for our purposes is that even if data sovereigns delegate power and authority to representatives and trustees, suspend their own authority through novel consent mechanisms, or renounce authority through blanket consent, some ethical constraints still remain in place. For example, individuals who upload their genome on OpenSNP do not thereby become fair game. Despite their broad consent, we can still raise questions about which use of their data is legitimate. Such questions arise from an ethical, but also from a legal perspective, e.g., when we debate which ways of discriminating against data subjects are unlawful. And in cases where consent procedures are tied to mechanisms of representation, Butler's remark suggests that representatives might be authorized to speak on behalf of data subjects, but can fail to articulate their voice. In some instances, the authority of representatives might "dissolve". These points illustrate that it remains an open and pressing question what researchers and data collectors owe to 'information altruists' and others who suspend their claims to full-fledged control over future use. The mere broadening of consent forms is not a surrogate for reflecting upon responsible institutional designs.

3.5.5 *Observation II*

There is considerable variation across the mentioned consent and representation models with regards to how well they cohere with the idea of a data *donation*. For example, in the above-mentioned picture of *collegial* research by Shirk et al., there is a sense in which data subjects are not donating any data *at all*. Their data does not go anywhere. It is merely channelled into a research process which the subjects themselves are designing and carrying out.

Broad consent might secure a link between self-determination and the process of sharing and subsequent analysis of personal health data. But here, some of the earlier challenges strike back. Precisely because the consent is broad, questions arise about how the apparent donor can meaningfully *endow* her data. After all, crucial aspects of her donation must remain open, including what exactly it is for, who benefits from it, and whether only she carries burdens related to the donation.

Tiered consent to data sharing, i.e. donating data towards specific purposes and/or with re-consent conditions in place, need not be strictly incompatible with the idea of a donation. But notice how when being provided by means of tiered consent, data is not simply *given* to others—researchers, developers, or the general public.

Instead, claims to power remain attached to it, and are not renounced by the apparent donor. Similar points apply to trustee or honest broker models. One of their purposes seems to be the extension of the donor's will to future situations and applications she cannot foresee in the present. These mechanisms allow the apparent donor to remain in command, if only indirectly and through representation, to ensure that use fits intended purpose. To put it bluntly: it is a little odd to make a donation or gift, but to tell recipients what to do with it. This request is driven to the maximum with dynamic consent, where the subject never actually ceases to be in control. All these mechanisms and models certainly hold alluring promises with regards to the protection and autonomy of individuals. But the question arises whether the apparent donor is actually put into a position where she clings onto what she has promised to let go off when entertaining and committing to the idea of a genuine data *donation*.

Taken together, the foregoing results lead to a puzzle. If I am giving some broad form of consent to use my personal health data, I lose my grip on the sense of endowment which authors like Mauss, Derrida, Ricœur, and Hénaff highlight as a distinctive feature of gifts. If I cling onto my data through various models of extending my control, I am not actually letting go.

Part of the puzzle might depend on the extent to which we regard donations as being more than exchange. It appears that all the aforementioned conditions are suitable means for the individual to retain power and control over her data and to constrain access and use it when this process is thought of as an exchange whose conditions the individual seeks to govern. But earlier (2.), we were suspecting that when being considered through the lens of gift theory, donations can be seen to exceed this logic, to point to something beyond economic exchange, and involve the acceptance of risks and uncertainties about the consequences of their endowment. If so, there is a tension between conditions to facilitate data donations as exercise of data sovereignty—in particular the resulting claims to power and control—and the idea of what it means to donate, gift, and endow something to others.

At this juncture, several strands of the foregoing discussion flow together. Data donations can reinforce the social structures in which individuals live their lives (2.). Specifically, data donations allow the individual to enact solidarity, beneficence, and participation (3.). Exercises of data sovereignty will thus not categorically result in restrictions to data access. Privacy must be ensured by default, but respecting individuals as data sovereigns further involves implementing responsible governance mechanisms to enable data donations. As we have seen, sovereignty is being realized through power and control. Data sovereignty in particular involves control over one's data: where it goes, who has access, and what is being done with it. Such control matters especially in view of the challenges and puzzles surrounding data donations (4.). Hence the three governance areas proposed above. However, on the one hand, gifting involves endowing and donating means letting go of what one gives. On the other hand, sovereignty involves power and control. The latter might undermine the former.

In view of this tension, should we not *refrain* from applying the sovereignty and gift paradigms, which we have claimed are inherently related, when trying to better understand the practice of data donations? Not necessarily. One intriguing way to resolve the tension just described is to regard data donations *as* data *loans*. When deciding whether or not to give an item, asset, or commodity, my options certainly include keeping all my claims to the object in place, i.e. not giving at all, *or* renouncing the entirety of my claims and giving without any remaining strings attached. But in between, a continuum of acts of giving is conceivable where only *some* kinds of claims to the object are renounced or suspended. Loans are instances where certain claims are being suspended and can be reclaimed at the conclusion of the loan (on the significance of this picture for understanding public attitudes towards scientific research, cf. Starkbaum et al. 2015; Braun and Dabrock 2016b). Other claims can remain in place throughout, e.g., when there are expectations about the purpose of the loan. As this illustrates, it is not inconsistent to give while keeping certain claims to the item, asset, or commodity in place. Loans as well as donations are something the lender gives, and her aims can include conveying recognition, fostering bonds of solidarity, and reinforcing social structures.

In our context, providing one's data to researchers need not be seen as a donation of the data itself. What is being given, potentially with all the aspects of endowment aspects described earlier (2., 3.), is a *loan* of this data. Individuals might want to retain certain powers, for example the ability to cancel or modify access if the challenges and evolving circumstances described earlier (4.) increase precarity or shift the nature of their data loan. If the motivation is genuinely non-self-interested, the loan carries no economic interest or benefit, no expected return in the light of which the lender's action pays off for her, other than putting her in a position to offer symbolic appreciation and contributions to others, her community, the scientific enterprise, and society as a whole. As an exercise of sovereignty, the loan comes with only one condition: that it may be retracted or at least the consent be modified if and when the individual requests it.

The picture of data donations *as* data loans does not resolve all challenges. Loans emphasize the precarious aspects of donations as they carry risks of exploitation and default. Lenders might strive in vain for control and security. Moreover, the question remains how individuals can lend something that they do not own in a straightforward way, and give a loan that in view of penetrative data processing is incredibly invasive. Nevertheless, the appeal of the picture is that it reflects both the ability to grant access to data and the implementation and justification of control mechanisms such as those outlined above. The latter might remain imperfect, but still be promising enough to set the wheel of giving in motion.

3.6 Conclusion

We have defended the thesis that donations of personal health data can advance individual sovereignty. The elements of gift theory have been used as a descriptive heuristic to gain a better understanding of donations. Gift theorists maintain that there are cases in which an analysis that focuses solely on *exchange* aspects elides important features of the target phenomenon. Instead, they invite us to look for what Derrida calls *aneconomic* aspects in order to grasp acts of giving in all their complexity: whether or not these acts involve a sense of endowment, are being carried out without the intention to prompt a return, transcend the individual's self-interest, and/or convey a symbolic, non-commodifiable aspect that encodes the donor's dedication and investment of a part of *herself* into what she is giving. Note that these suggestions are *descriptive*. It does not follow that it is normatively desirable to make gifts, just that considering these aspects ameliorates our understanding of acts of giving.

Once donations are examined through the lens of gift theory, it becomes apparent that they can generate social bonds, convey recognition and open up new options in social space, for example by interrupting patterns of economic exchange and enabling activities and interactions that would have otherwise remained unlikely or impossible. If these potentials are realized, donations can be fruitful advances of individual sovereignty. Sovereignty is sometimes being reduced to negative and protective rights and powers, but we suggested that it also encompasses positive entitlements to pursue one's notion of the good life through connecting and interacting with others. Our claim was not that donations are the only way to advance sovereignty. However, if data subjects are to be sovereigns about their health data, the positive dimension of sovereignty calls for ways to *facilitate* the sharing of data as an expression of the individual's informational self-determination. Such donations can enact solidarity and beneficence and enable donors to participate in scientific processes.

The foregoing neither motivates a duty to donate nor deflates the importance of protections. Even though donations can advance positive sovereignty, we must not lose sight of potential *conflicts* with the negative, protective aspects of sovereignty. Data donations in particular have a range of features that exacerbate risks and uncertainties. In big data contexts, data donations become more invasive than other kinds of donations. Potential data donors are bound to have a limited grip on what they are giving, the future use of their data, and the people affected by their decision to share.

We thus proposed that tensions between data donations and the negative, protective aspects of sovereignty shall be minimized through consent procedures, the representation of data subjects, and organization-level constraints and commitments. These mechanisms complement one another and apply to a plurality of agents on different levels (Braun and Dabrock 2016a, pp. 324–5; German Ethics Council 2017a, sect. 5.3): individuals who become empowered to share and withdraw their data, representatives and brokers who mediate between individuals and data processors, data networks which provide means for data subjects to govern the flow of their information, and regulators who set formal and enforceable frameworks. These mechanisms seek to ensure the *controllability* of data donations for individuals as well as the *accountability* of data gatherers and processors. Ideally, the intentions of data donors, including those related to gifting and endowing, can then be introduced and unfold within the governance of the institution.

Special attention should be paid to technological infrastructures. First, data interoperability (Nature Biotechnology 2015) is necessary to transfer data, e.g., from electronic health records or direct-to-consumer genetic testing to data networks. Second, our call for dynamic consent mechanisms requires user-friendly interfaces in order to make users aware of new developments and allow them to control, submit, and withdraw data in real-time. Third, developing such interfaces and/or setting up representatives, typically software data agents, to serve as data trustees presupposes a sufficient degree of standardization of programmatic data interfaces.

Nevertheless, in the end all these measures might fall short. Recall Derrida's claim that gifts set the circle of the economy in motion. We can set up efficient infrastructures and implement *controllability* for donors as well as *accountability* of data-processing institutions. Still, Derrida's claim can be taken to remind us that institutions of giving will be set in motion only if individuals are ready to engage in this risky enterprise—an enterprise that opens up opportunities, but in which frustrations and harms can never be ruled out. That is, a particular kind of endowment is required: individuals need to *trust* and engage in the act of giving despite the risk that it will not have its intended effects. This is not a normative demand that potential donors shall trust the system that seeks their contribution. The claim is, again, descriptive: trust is what sets the system in motion, and if trust is lost, everything comes to a halt. This insight is perfectly compatible with the further claim that *once* donors trust and decide to give, mechanisms that implement accountability, controllability as well as norms of transparency remain indispensable to keep the process functional and sustainable. The necessity of such momentums of endowment highlights a strength of gift theory: it helps us to discern certain *aneconomic* working principles of our institutions that might have otherwise escaped our attention.

If the donor transfers authority over her data by means of broad consent, it becomes hard to get a grip on future uses and beneficiaries, which appears to be in tension with the idea of meaningfully endowing such data. If consent is dynamic or tiered, one is not actually letting go of what one appears to donate, and thus deflates the sense in which one makes a genuine donation. These observations could be seen as reasons to *refrain* from applying the gift paradigm to data donations. However, we have argued for a different approach. Data donations—at least those that are cognizant of the claims of sovereign individuals—come in a particular form: unlike other forms of donation, they are most plausibly understood as *loans* rather than *transfers*.

Acknowledgments We are grateful for funding from the German Federal Ministry of Health (ZMV/1 – 2517 FSB 013).

References

23andMe. 2018. Becoming part of something bigger. https://www.23andme.com/en-int/research/. Accessed 31 Jan 2018.

Ajana, B. 2018. Communal self-tracking: Data philanthropy, solidarity and privacy. In *Self-tracking*, ed. B. Ajana, 125–141. Cham: Palgrave Macmillan. https://doi.org/10.1007/978-3-319-65379-2_9.

Baylis, F., N.P. Kenny, and S. Sherwin. 2008. A relational account of public health ethics. *Public Health Ethics* 1 (3): 196–209. https://doi.org/10.1093/phe/phn025.

Berliner, L.S., and N.J. Kenworthy. 2017. Producing a worthy illness: Personal crowdfunding amidst financial crisis. *Social Science & Medicine (1982)* 187: 233–242. https://doi.org/10.1016/j.socscimed.2017.02.008.

Bialobrzeski, A., J. Ried, and P. Dabrock. 2012. Differentiating and evaluating common good and public good: Making implicit assumptions explicit in the contexts of consent and duty to participate. *Public Health Genomics* 15 (5): 285–292. https://doi.org/10.1159/000336861.

Bodin, J. 1576. *On sovereignty. Four chapters from six books of the commonwealth*, ed. J.H. Franklin. Cambridge: Cambridge University Press 1992.

Borgman, C.L. 2012. The conundrum of sharing research data. *Journal of the American Society for Information Science and Technology* 63 (6): 1059–1078. https://doi.org/10.1002/asi.22634.

Braun, M. 2017. *Zwang und Anerkennung*. Tübingen: Mohr-Siebeck.

Braun, M., and P. Dabrock. 2016a. Ethische Herausforderungen einer sogenannten Big-Data basierten Medizin. *Zeitschrift für medizinische Ethik, 4/*2016.

———. 2016b. 'I bet you won't': The science-society wager on gene editing techniques. *EMBO Reports* 17 (3): 279–280. https://doi.org/10.15252/embr.201541935.

Butler, J. 2015. *Notes toward a performative theory of assembly*. Harvard: Harvard University Press.

Cargill, S.S. 2016. Biobanking and the abandonment of informed consent: An ethical imperative. *Public Health Ethics* 9 (3): 255–263. https://doi.org/10.1093/phe/phw001.

Caulfield, T., R.E. Upshur, and A. Daar. 2003. DNA databanks and consent: A suggested policy option involving an authorization model. *BMC Medical Ethics* 4 (1). https://doi.org/10.1186/1472-6939-4-1.

Dabrock, P. 2012. *Befähigungsgerechtigkeit. Ein Grundkonzept konkreter Ethik in fundamental-theologischer Perspektive*. Gütersloh: Gütersloher Verlagshaus.

———. 2018. Die Würde des Menschen ist granularisierbar. Muss die Grundlage unseres Gemeinwesens neu gedacht werden? *epd-Dokumentation* 22 (18): 8–16.

Dabrock, P., L. Klinnert, and S. Schardien. 2004. *Menschenwürde und Lebensschutz: Herausforderungen theologischer Bioethik*. Gütersloh: Gütersloher Verlagshaus.

De Filippi, P., and S. McCarthy. 2012. Cloud computing: Centralization and data sovereignty. *European Journal of Law and Technology* 3 (2). http://ejlt.org/article/view/101/245. Accessed 12 Apr 2018.

De Mooy, M. 2017. *Rethinking privacy self-management and data sovereignty in the age of big data: Considerations for future policy regimes in the United States and the European Union*. Gütersloh: Bertelsmann Stiftung.

de Mul, J. 2014. Artificial by nature. An introduction to Plessner's philosophical anthropology. In *Plessner's philosophical anthropology*, ed. J. de Mul. Amsterdam: Amsterdam University Press.

Derrida, J. 1992. *Given time: I. counterfeit money*. (trans: Kamuf, P.). Chicago: University of Chicago Press.

DNA.Land. 2018. DNA.Land. Know Your Genome. Help Science. https://dna.land/

Eiseman, E., G. Bloom, J. Brower, N. Clancy, and S.S. Olmsted. 2003. *Case studies of existing human tissue repositories: 'Best Practices' for a biospecimen resource for the genomic and proteomic era*. Santa Monica: Rand Corporation.

Foucault, M. 1977. *Discipline and punish: The birth of the prison*. 1995th ed. New York: Vintage Books.

Fox, R.C., and J.P. Swazey. 1978. *The courage to fail: A social view of organ transplants and dialysis*. London and New York: Routledge 2017.

Friedrichsen, M., and P.-J. Bisa. 2016. *Digitale Souveränität: Vertrauen in der Netzwerkgesellschaft*. Wiesbaden: Springer.

Gent, E. 2017. Our health data can save lives, but we have to be willing to share. https://singularityhub.com/2017/02/16/our-health-data-can-save-lives-but-we-have-to-be-willing-to-share/?utm_source=Singularity+Hub+Newsletter&utm_campaign=a88276628c-Hub_Daily_Newsletter&utm_medium=email&utm_term=0_f0cf60cdae-a88276628c-58134781

German Ethics Council. 2017a. *Big data and health. Data sovereignty as the shaping of informational freedom (Executive Summary & Recommendations)*. Berlin: German Ethics Council. https://www.ethikrat.org/fileadmin/Publikationen/Stellungnahmen/englisch/opinion-big-data-and-health-summary.pdf. Accessed 9 Feb 2018.

———. 2017b. *Big Data und Gesundheit. Datensouveränität als informationelle Freiheitsgestaltung*. Berlin: German Ethics Council. https://www.ethikrat.org/fileadmin/Publikationen/Stellungnahmen/deutsch/stellungnahme-big-data-und-gesundheit.pdf. Accessed 9 Feb 2018.

Gill, P., and L. Lowes. 2008. Gift exchange and organ donation: Donor and recipient experiences of live related kidney transplantation. *International Journal of Nursing Studies* 45: 1607–1617.

Goodman, B. 2016. What's wrong with the right to genetic privacy: Beyond exceptionalism, parochialism and adventitious ethics. In *The ethics of biomedical big data*, ed. B.D. Mittelstadt and L. Floridi, 139–167. Cham: Springer. https://doi.org/10.1007/978-3-319-33525-4_7.

Grajales, F., D. Clifford, P. Loupos, S. Okun, S. Quattrone, M. Simon, et al. 2014. Social networking sites and the continuously learning health system: A survey. Institute of Medicine of the National Academies. https://nam.edu/wp-content/uploads/2015/06/VSRT-PatientDataSharing.pdf. Accessed 27 Jan 2018.

Harari, Y.N. 2016. *Homo Deus. A brief history of tomorrow*. New York: Harper.

Hayden, E.C. 2012. A broken contract. *Nature* (486). https://www.nature.com/polopoly_fs/1.10862!/menu/main/topColumns/topLeftColumn/pdf/486312a.pdf?origin=ppub. Accessed 9 Feb 2018.

———. 2015. Proposed Ebola biobank would strengthen African science. *Nature News* 524 (7564): 146. https://doi.org/10.1038/524146a.

Health Data Exploration Project. 2014. Personal data for the public good: New opportunities to enrich understanding of individual and population health. California Institute for Telecommunications and Information Technology. http://hdexplore.calit2.net/wp-content/uploads/2015/08/hdx_final_report_small.pdf.

Hénaff, M. 2010. The Price of truth: Gift, money, and philosophy. (trans: Morhange, J.-L.). Stanford: Stanford University Press.

———. 2013. Ceremonial gift-giving: The lessons of anthropology from mauss and beyond. In *The gift in antiquity*, ed. M.L. Satlow, 12–24. Chichester: Wiley-Blackwell.

Hobbes, T. 1651. *Leviathan*, ed. R. Tuck. Cambridge: Cambridge University Press 1996.

Hornung, G., and C. Schnabel. 2009. Data protection in Germany I: The population census decision and the right to informational self-determination. *Computer Law & Security Review* 25 (1): 84–88. https://doi.org/10.1016/j.clsr.2008.11.002.

International Covenant on Economic, Social and Cultural Rights. 1966. http://www.ohchr.org/Documents/ProfessionalInterest/cescr.pdf

Ioannidis, J.P.A. 2013. Informed consent, big data, and the oxymoron of research that is not research. *The American Journal of Bioethics* 13 (4): 40–42. https://doi.org/10.1080/15265161.2013.768864.

Irion, K. 2013. Government cloud computing and national data sovereignty. *Policy & Internet* 4 (3–4): 40–71. https://doi.org/10.1002/poi3.10.

Kant, I. (1785). In *Groundwork of the metaphysics of morals*, ed. M. Gregor and J. Timmermann. Cambridge: Cambridge University Press 2011.

Kirkpatrick, R. 2011. Data philanthropy: Public & private sector data sharing for global resilience. *United Nations Global Pulse*. https://www.unglobalpulse.org/blog/data-philanthropy-public-private-sector-data-sharing-global-resilience. Accessed 27 Jan 2018.

———. 2013, March 21. A new type of philanthropy: Donating data. *Harvard Business Review*. https://hbr.org/2013/03/a-new-type-of-philanthropy-don. Accessed 16 Feb 2018.

Knoppers, B.M., J.R. Harris, I. Budin-Ljøsne, and E.S. Dove. 2014. A human rights approach to an international code of conduct for genomic and clinical data sharing. *Human Genetics* 133 (7): 895–903. https://doi.org/10.1007/s00439-014-1432-6.

Kohane, I.S., and R.B. Altman. 2005. Health-information altruists — A potentially critical resource. *The New Englang Journal of Medicine* 353 (19): 2074–2077.

Kostkova, P., H. Brewer, S. de Lusignan, E. Fottrell, B. Goldacre, G. Hart, et al. 2016. Who owns the data? Open data for healthcare. *Frontiers in Public Health* 4. https://doi.org/10.3389/fpubh.2016.00007.

Krempl, S. 2018. Datensouveränität: Die Säge am informationellen Selbstbestimmungsrecht. *heise online*. https://www.heise.de/newsticker/meldung/Datensouveraenitaet-Die-Saege-am-informationellen-Selbstbestimmungsrecht-3953776.html. Accessed 13 Aug 2018.

MacAskill, W. 2015. *Doing good better: Effective altruism and a radical new way to make a difference*. London: Guardian Faber Publishing.

Mackenzie, C., and N. Stoljar. 2000. *Relational autonomy: Feminist perspectives on autonomy, agency, and the social self*. Oxford: Oxford University Press.

Maritain, J. 1951. *Man and the state*. Chicago: Chicago Universit Press 1998.

Master, Z., L. Campo-Engelstein, and T. Caulfield. 2015. Scientists' perspectives on consent in the context of biobanking research. *European Journal of Human Genetics* 23 (5): 569–574. https://doi.org/10.1038/ejhg.2014.143.

Mauss, M. 1950. *The gift. The form and reason for exchange in archaic societies*. London and New York: Routledge 2002.

Mayer-Schönberger, V., and K. Cukier. 2013. *Big data: A revolution that will transform how we live, work, and think*. Boston: Houghton Mifflin Harcourt.

Microsoft. 2018. Project InnerEye – Medical imaging AI to empower clinicians. *Microsoft Research*. https://www.microsoft.com/en-us/research/project/medical-image-analysis/.

Mill, J.S. 1859. On liberty. In *The collected works of John Stuart Mill, vol. XVIII*, ed. J.M. Robson. Toronto: Toronto University Press 2008.

Mittelstadt, B.D., and L. Floridi. 2016. The ethics of big data: Current and foreseeable issues in biomedical contexts. In *The ethics of biomedical big data*, 445–480. Cham: Springer. https://doi.org/10.1007/978-3-319-33525-4_19.

Montgomery, J. 2017. Data sharing and the idea of ownership. *The New Bioethics* 23 (1): 81–86. https://doi.org/10.1080/20502877.2017.1314893.

Murdoch, T.B., and A.S. Detsky. 2013. The inevitable application of big data to health care. *JAMA* 309 (13): 1351–1352. https://doi.org/10.1001/jama.2013.393.

Nature Biotechnology. 2015. Incentivizing data donation. *Nature Biotechnology* 33 (9): 885. https://doi.org/10.1038/nbt.3341.

Nuffield Council on Bioethics. 2015. *The collection, linking and use of data in biomedical research and health care: Ethical issues*. Nuffield Council on Bioethics. http://nuffieldbioethics.org/wp-content/uploads/Biological_and_health_data_web.pdf. Accessed 9 Feb 2018.

PatientsLikeMe. 2014. PatientsLikeMe launches "Data for Good" campaign to encourage health data sharing to advance medicine. http://news.patientslikeme.com/press-release/patientslikeme-launches-data-good-campaign-encourage-health-data-sharing-advance-medic. Accessed 27 Jan 2018.

Peterson, Z.N.J., M. Gondree, and R. Beverly. 2011. A position paper on data sovereignty: The importance of geolocating data in the cloud. In *Proceedings of the 3rd USENIX conference on hot topics in cloud computing*. Berkeley: USENIX Association. https://www.usenix.org/legacy/events/hotcloud11/tech/final_files/Peterson.pdf. Accessed 12 Apr 2018.

Petrini, C. 2010. "Broad" consent, exceptions to consent and the question of using biological samples for research purposes different from the initial collection purpose. *Social Science & Medicine* 70 (2): 217–220. https://doi.org/10.1016/j.socscimed.2009.10.004.

Plessner, H. 1980. Die Stufen des Organischen und der Mensch. Einleitung in die philosophische Anthropologie. In *Gesammelte Schriften*, ed. G. Dux, vol. V. Frankfurt am Main: Suhrkamp.

Prainsack, B. 2018. The "We" in the "Me": Solidarity and health care in the era of personalized medicine. *Science, Technology, & Human Values* 43 (1): 21–44. https://doi.org/10.1177/0162243917736139.

Prainsack, B., and A. Buyx. 2012. Solidarity in contemporary bioethics — Towards a new approach. *Bioethics* 26 (7): 343–350. https://doi.org/10.1111/j.1467-8519.2012.01987.x.

———. 2017. *Solidarity in biomedicine and beyond*. Cambridge: Cambridge University Press.

Pummer, T. 2016. Whether and where to give. *Philosophy & Public Affairs* 44 (1): 77–95.

Raghupathi, W., and V. Raghupathi. 2014. Big data analytics in healthcare: Promise and potential. *Health Information Science and Systems* 2: 3. https://doi.org/10.1186/2047-2501-2-3.

Ricœur, P. 2005. *The course of recognition*. Harvard: Harvard University Press.

Schapranow, M.-P., J. Brauer, and H. Plattner. 2017. The data donation pass: Enabling sovereign control of personal healthcare data. In *Proceedings of the 2017 international conference on Health Informatics and Medical Systems (HIMS'17)*. Las Vegas: CSREA Press.

Sharon, T. 2017. Self-tracking for health and the quantified self: Re-articulating autonomy, solidarity, and authenticity in an age of personalized healthcare. *Philosophy & Technology* 30 (1): 93–121. https://doi.org/10.1007/s13347-016-0215-5.

Shirk, J.L., H.L. Ballard, C.C. Wilderman, T. Phillips, A. Wiggins, R. Jordan, et al. 2012. Public participation in scientific research: A framework for deliberate design. *Ecology and Society* 17 (2). http://www.jstor.org/stable/26269051. Accessed 1 Mar 2018.

Simpson, B. 2018. A 'we' problem for bioethics and the social sciences: A response to Barbara Prainsack. *Science, Technology, & Human Values* 43 (1): 45–55. https://doi.org/10.1177/0162243917735899.

Singer, P. 2009. *The life you can save*. New York: Random House.

———. 2015. *The most good you can do. How effective altruism is changing ideas about living ethically*. New Haven and London: Yale University Press.

Snyder, J. 2016. Crowdfunding for medical care: Ethical issues in an emerging health care funding practice. *The Hastings Center Report* 46 (6): 36–42. https://doi.org/10.1002/hast.645.

Sque, M., and S.A. Payne. 1994. Gift exchange theory: A critique in relation to organ transplantation. *Journal of Advanced Nursing* 19 (1): 45–51. https://doi.org/10.1111/j.1365-2648.1994.tb01049.x.

Starkbaum, J., M. Braun, and P. Dabrock. 2015. The synthetic biology puzzle: A qualitative study on public reflections towards a governance framework. *Systems and Synthetic Biology* 9: 147–157. https://doi.org/10.1007/s11693-015-9182-x.

Steinfath, H., and C. Wiesemann, eds. 2016. *Autonomie und Vertrauen: Schlüsselbegriffe der modernen Medizin*. Wiesbaden: Springer VS.

Sterckx, S., J. Cockbain, H.C. Howard, and P. Borry. 2013, October 3. "I prefer a child with …": Designer babies, another controversial patent in the arena of direct-to-consumer genomics. *Genetics in Medicine*. Comments and Opinion. https://doi.org/10.1038/gim.2013.164.

Sterckx, S., V. Rakic, J. Cockbain, and P. Borry. 2016. "You hoped we would sleep walk into accepting the collection of our data": Controversies surrounding the UK care.Data scheme and their wider relevance for biomedical research. *Medicine, Health Care and Philosophy* 19 (2): 177–190. https://doi.org/10.1007/s11019-015-9661-6.

Taylor, C. 1985. *Philosophical papers: Volume 2, philosophy and the human sciences*. Cambridge: Cambridge University Press.

The Council for International Organizations of Medical Sciences (CIOMS). 2016. *International ethical guidelines for biomedical research involving human subjects*. Geneva: Council for International Organizations of Medical Sciences (CIOMS).

Universal Declaration of Human Rights. 1948. http://www.un.org/en/universal-declaration-human-rights/.

Vaught, J., and N.C. Lockhart. 2012. The evolution of biobanking best practices. *Clinica Chimica Acta* 413 (19): 1569–1575. https://doi.org/10.1016/j.cca.2012.04.030.

Vayena, E., and A. Blasimme. 2017. Biomedical big data: New models of control over access, use and governance. *Journal of Bioethical Inquiry* 14 (4): 501–513. https://doi.org/10.1007/s11673-017-9809-6.

Vayena, E., and J. Tasioulas. 2015. "We the scientists": A human right to citizen science. *Philosophy & Technology* 28 (3): 479–485. https://doi.org/10.1007/s13347-015-0204-0.

———. 2016. The dynamics of big data and human rights: The case of scientific research. *Philosophical Transactions of the Royal Society A* 374 (2083). https://doi.org/10.1098/rsta.2016.0129.

Vayena, E., M. Salathé, L.C. Madoff, and J.S. Brownstein. 2015. Ethical challenges of big data in public health. *PLoS Computational Biology* 11 (2): e1003904. https://doi.org/10.1371/journal.pcbi.1003904.

Vernale, G., and Packard. 1990. Organ donation as gift exchange. *The Journal of Nursing Scholarship* 22 (4): 239–242. https://doi.org/10.1111/j.1547-5069.1990.tb00221.x.

Waldenfels, B. 2012. *Hyperphänomene: Modi hyperbolischer Erfahrung*. Frankfurt: Suhrkamp.

Weitzman, E.R., L. Kaci, and K.D. Mandl. 2010. Sharing medical data for health research: The early personal health record experience. *Journal of Medical Internet Research* 12 (2): e14. https://doi.org/10.2196/jmir.1356.

Wellcome Trust. 2013. Summary report of qualitative research into public attitudes to personal data and linking personal data: *Wellcome Library*. http://wellcomelibrary.org/item/b20997358. Accessed 9 Feb 2018.

World Health Organization. 2015. WHO First Consultation on Ebola Biobanking. *WHO*. http://www.who.int/medicines/ebola-treatment/1st_consult_ebola_biobank/en/. Accessed 9 Feb 2018.

World Medical Association. 1964. Ethical principles for medical research involving human subjects. https://www.wma.net/policies-post/wma-declaration-of-helsinki-ethical-principles-for-medical-research-involving-human-subjects/. Accessed 9 Feb 2018.

Yang, Y., P.A. Fasching, M. Wallwiener, T.N. Fehm, S.Y. Brucker, and V. Tresp. 2016. Predictive clinical decision support system with RNN encoding and tensor decoding. In *arXiv:1612.00611 [cs]*. http://arxiv.org/abs/1612.00611. Accessed 25 Feb 2018.

Yang, Y., P.A. Fasching, and V. Tresp. 2017. Predictive modeling of therapy decisions in metastatic breast cancer with recurrent neural network encoder and multinomial hierarchical regression decoder. In *2017 IEEE International Conference on Healthcare Informatics (ICHI)* (pp. 46–55). Presented at the 2017 IEEE international conference on healthcare informatics (ICHI). https://doi.org/10.1109/ICHI.2017.51.

Yassin, R., N. Lockhart, M. del González Riego, K. Pitt, J.W. Thomas, L. Weiss, and C. Compton. 2010. Custodianship as an ethical framework for biospecimen-based research. *Cancer Epidemiology, Biomarkers & Prevention* 19 (4): 1012–1015. https://doi.org/10.1158/1055-9965.EPI-10-0029.

Chapter 4
The Ethics of Uncertainty for Data Subjects

Philip J. Nickel

Abstract Modern health data practices come with many practical uncertainties. In this paper, I argue that data subjects' trust in the institutions and organizations that control their data, and their ability to know their own moral obligations in relation to their data, are undermined by significant uncertainties regarding the what, how, and who of mass data collection and analysis. I conclude by considering how proposals for managing situations of high uncertainty might be applied to this problem. These emphasize increasing organizational flexibility, knowledge, and capacity, and reducing hazard.

Keywords Ethics of data donation · Practical uncertainty · Opacity of algorithms · Profiling · Trust · Value-based health care · Systemic oversight · Privacy-by-design · Data professionalism

4.1 Uncertainty and Data Ethics

Modern mass data collection and analysis promise great innovation in the health domain, as well as significant uncertainty. The CEO of one of the world's largest technology companies has said that "fear of data-mining" leads to 100,000 preventable deaths per year (Hern 2014). One plausible explanation for such fear is that health data subjects feel uncertain about the implications of data innovation.

In this chapter the uncertainty surrounding emerging technologies is analyzed as a practical problem for data subjects. The style of ethical analysis employed here is somewhat new. Brey writes that "the main problem for the ethics of emerging technology is the problem of uncertainty"; however, in contrast to the present approach, he proposes "anticipatory technology ethics that tries to forecast various possible future developments" (Brey 2017, 175, 178). The analysis in this chapter is

P. J. Nickel (✉)
Eindhoven University of Technology, Eindhoven, The Netherlands
e-mail: p.j.nickel@tue.nl

J. Krutzinna, L. Floridi (eds.), *The Ethics of Medical Data Donation*,
Philosophical Studies Series 137, https://doi.org/10.1007/978-3-030-04363-6_4

complementary to such an "anticipatory ethics" but does not aim to forecast future developments. Instead, it looks at the causes and practical consequences of uncertainty for data subjects in the present tense.[1]

Some rough definitions of key concepts are needed for this analysis. *Practical uncertainties* are defined as things we *do not know* and have an *interest* in knowing (Goldman 1999; Fallis 2006). Their ethical significance therefore has two dimensions: (a) the features of data practices that create unknowns; and (b) the interests of data subjects that are impeded by these unknowns.

Data subjects refers to those people whose data is collected and processed, whether they provide this data voluntarily or not. For example, a person who gives access to genetic test results or uses 'wearable' or in-home medical data-collecting devices, or consumer smartphones with built-in health services is a data subject. In cases where people provide highly explicit and voluntary consent to the transfer of data, we can speak of *donation*. However, in what follows it will be argued that within the context of current data practices it is often unclear whether a data transfer can really count as a donation, because whether it is truly a donation is itself a morally significant uncertainty.

The argument here concerns health data but is also relevant for many other domains where personal data is shared and collected on a mass scale, such as social media, financial planning, workplaces, and urban spaces. The boundaries between health data and other kinds of personal data are blurring to some extent: "The traditional boundaries of primary and tertiary care environments are breaking down and health information is increasingly collected through mobile devices, in personal domains … and from sensors attached on or in the human body …. At the same time, the detail and diversity of information collected in the context of healthcare and biomedical research is increasing at an unprecedented rate" (Malin et al. 2013, 2). An extension of this point is that a great deal of not-seemingly-health-related data can be used for medical and health purposes (Prainsack 2017).

In accordance with the definition of practical uncertainty above, the argument to be pursued here can be expressed in the following way:

1. Fundamental features of our data practices, including the open-endedness of data to new insights and applications, the opacity of data analysis (here referring to the inaccessibility and/or incomprehensibility of how algorithms analyze data), and the persistence of data, imply uncertainty regarding the what, how, and who of data practices.
2. Two important epistemic interests of data subjects are threatened by this uncertainty: (i) having trust in the institutions that manage data, and (ii) knowing one's ethical obligations with respect to data sharing.
3. Therefore, other things equal, we should take feasible policy measures to mitigate uncertainty.

[1] In this sense, my approach is what Brey would label a "generic approach" to the ethics of emerging technology that considers "inherent features of the technology" rather than an "anticipatory approach" that uses "foresight methods" (op. cit., 178–179). However, it analyzes uncertainties *about* the future.

In line with this argument, Sect. 4.2 discusses some endemic aspects of our data practices that create uncertainties, and Sect. 4.3 addresses our interests in having knowledge in the domain of health data. Section 4.4 concerns possible strategies for mitigating uncertainty. Such strategies, if effective, could make it less ethically problematic to obtain the many benefits associated with mass data collection and analysis, and could help people overcome the "fear of data mining" mentioned at the beginning of this section.

4.2 What Features of Data Practices Create Unknowns?

Three features of data and data practices—*open-endedness*, *opacity*, and *persistence*—together give rise to significant uncertainties for data subjects. These uncertainties are distinctive because they cannot easily be avoided by engaging in best practices for risk reduction (for example, through better data security). To some extent they are part and parcel of any scenario for mass collection and processing of data. They are not futuristic. They are implied by many practitioners' statements about current practices, both routine and avant-garde, as well as in current interpretation of these practices. Those familiar with data ethics might find the features of data practices discussed in what follows unsurprising. What is new here is how they are conceptualized and deployed in relation to uncertainty. The focus is on uncertainties that arise, not only when something goes wrong with the management of data, but also when it is being used as its controllers intend: uncertainties due to the very nature of digital data as a form of information and our practices of using it.[2]

Before exploring these three uncertainty-creating characteristics of modern data practices, a brief remark is needed about what uncertainty means here. In practical ethics we are often concerned with *risky* uncertainties: possible, unwanted future states of affairs (e.g., possible data thefts). Risk and uncertainty are often defined so that they refer to distinct phenomena: 'risk proper' is probabilistic uncertainty about future unwanted events where both the probabilities and the possible outcomes of these events are known and quantifiable, whereas 'uncertainty proper' is a lack of knowledge about which outcomes are possible and/or their probabilities (Knight 1921; cf. Altham 1983). Some authors draw a further distinction between uncertainty and ignorance, where ignorance involves inability to predict outcomes or plausible scenarios (Wynne 1992, cited in Dereli et al. 2014). The kind of uncertainty to be discussed in what follows lies in between the categories of uncertainty proper and ignorance: we can identify some plausible horizons of possibility, but not exhaustively or quantifiably.[3]

[2] Collingridge (1980) is famous for arguing that we can only control the risks of technological innovation early in its development, but we can only know what risks to try to prevent after it is well underway. The uncertainties I focus on here cannot easily be prevented for another reason, which is that they are almost inseparable from the underlying data practices, strongly linked with the transformative potential of those practices, and therefore not likely to be eliminated.

[3] Consequences known to be harmful for some individuals are likely to be directly caused by the further development of big data practices, such as the ability to reidentify unidentified ("anony-

4.2.1 Open-Endedness

Open-endedness—the potential for creating and applying data-based knowledge in new ways—creates significant uncertainties for data subjects at the time when their data is collected and afterwards. Data is multiply interpretable, especially when combined and used for new purposes. Different algorithms and analytical lenses, such as different strategies of classifying, combining, and finding patterns in data, allow for new predictions and correlative generalizations. This is essential to the promises of data collection and analysis: "the value of big data lies in the unexpectedness of the insights that it can reveal" (Barocas and Nissenbaum 2014, 60). Since we cannot form expectations about these important insights, open-endedness creates significant uncertainties.

There are at least two dimensions of open-endedness. The first is the *fecundity* of inferences that can be drawn when a dataset is larger or better organized, or where more powerful analytical tools are used. The second is *recontextualization* of data across contexts. We can think of the first dimension as the *depth or power* of the inferences we can make from a set of data, and the second dimension as the *practical applicability* of these inferences in a diverse range of contexts in real time.[4]

A real-life example of open-endedness from the health domain is the vision of the 'value-based health care' movement. This movement proposes to align payment for health services closely with actual health outcomes, creating a transformation of health care. Its founders have maintained from the beginning that data collection and analysis are necessary instruments for this transition because they make it possible to develop and apply a nuanced health-improvement metric for reimbursing health costs across the board. One early proponent, focusing on the inefficiencies of the American health care system, devotes several paragraphs to the importance of data as a means toward value-based care:

> Measurement and dissemination of health outcomes should become mandatory for every provider and every medical condition … We need to measure true health outcomes rather than relying solely on process measures, such as compliance with practice guidelines, which are incomplete and slow to change. … Among our highest near-term priorities is to finalize and then continuously update health information technology (HIT) standards that include precise data definitions (for diagnoses and treatments, for example), an architecture

mous") data subjects using new and more powerful analytical techniques. This could in some cases lead to loss of insurance or other harms for re-identified individuals. For example, in Lippert et al.'s (2017) controversial study, recognizable images of the faces of individuals were said to be reconstructable using data from gene sequences. There is dispute about whether the results really prove what the authors say (Erlich 2017). Irrespective of this dispute, my point here is that the looming possibility of such techniques creates horizons of uncertainty that exist long before any future harms that result. These uncertainties are ethically significant in their own right.

[4] Some commentators have raised epistemological concerns that big data is overhyped as a scientific field and may not withstand scientific scrutiny of its knowledge claims (Mittelstadt and Floridi 2016; Lipworth et al. 2017). My argument does not depend on the validity of the relevant knowledge claims as a whole, but rather their plausibility.

> for aggregating data for each patient over time and across providers, and protocols for seamless communication among systems (Porter 2009).

This underlying idea has persisted both in value-based health care and in other similar movements such as the Institute of Medicine's 'learning health care system': with new sources of data and analytical tools, we can explore new ways of modeling and addressing the causes of inefficiency and suboptimal health outcomes (Committee 2013; Mulley et al. 2017). Both fecundity of insight *and* recontextualization of real-time decision-making are needed for the envisioned transformations.

Other examples emphasize recontextualization to a greater degree: cases in which an integrated situational awareness is stitched together from data originating in multiple contexts, creating a single 'dashboard' or 'visualization' for decision-making. Suppose two large sets of data on treatments, costs, and patient outcomes, one collected by hospitals, and a second collected by general practitioners, are being combined for the first time. If health care is managed through substantially separate structures, then mutual access to this information holds the prospect of bringing about better integration and continuity of health care for both hospitals and GPs (e.g., Sheaff et al. 2015, 57). Similar contextual awareness is anticipated elsewhere in health care: for example, in the integration of "informal health and fitness data collected by the user together with official health records collected by health professionals" (Gay and Leijdekkers 2015). These cases stress the recontextualization of information, but also promise insight when complementary data is combined.

Profiling people in multiple and unpredictable ways is an ethically relevant aspect of open-endedness in data analysis. Profiling has been defined as "the process of 'discovering' patterns in data … that can be used to identify or represent a human or nonhuman subject (individual or group) and/or the application of profiles (sets of correlated data) to individuate and represent an individual subject or to identify a subject as a member of a group (which can be an existing community or a discovered category)" (Hildebrandt 2009, 275). This and other definitions explicitly relate to both dimensions of open-endedness: fecundity ("discovering") and recontextualization ("application", "identification"). Profiling is particularly relevant to data subjects in a health context because it has the potential to classify them for diagnosis, treatment, and reimbursement in unpredictable ways. For example, it might be used as a reason to choose a particular diagnostic, or to deny treatment altogether.

4.2.2 Opacity

A second source of endemic uncertainty in our data practices is the use of opaque algorithms and 'deep learning' to analyze data (Kennedy et al. 2015; Rieder and Simon 2017). Consider a widely discussed recent example in which a deep learning algorithm was trained to identify profile photos from a prominent social media site as being gay/lesbian or straight (Wang and Kosinski 2018). The algorithm was able to determine this with considerable accuracy, better than that of human raters. However, because the training was automatic and data-driven, it is not known what features the machine correlated with sexual orientation identity.

This example shows that one possible reason why data analytics is opaque is that deep learning techniques do not disclose the underlying pattern of their learning (Mittelstadt et al. 2016). Some algorithms are highly complex, and some are modified frequently (Rieder and Simon 2017, 6). However, not all algorithms are complex or difficult to understand; there are also other reasons why data analytics is opaque. One is secrecy: algorithms are often not shared due to intellectual property issues, competitiveness, inertia, or concerns that they will not withstand scrutiny (Burrell 2016; Christophersen et al. 2015; Gillingham 2016; Stodden 2010).

A complicating issue is that data subjects rarely have the concepts needed to understand the actual algorithms and deep learning techniques themselves. However, that is not in itself an epistemological barrier to knowledge. On many views of knowledge in a social world, it is socially constituted. Laypeople can have knowledge that is partly constituted by the knowledge and understanding of others, including experts (Faulkner 2011; Goldberg 2010). A serious problem arises principally when experts do not have this knowledge themselves, *or* when they do not carry out their functions in a way that confers socially constituted knowledge upon data subjects. For example, a plausible condition on socially constituted knowledge is that there is some person or collective of persons that has understanding and is willing and able to provide an articulate explanation when asked or challenged.[5] When trained scientists working with opaque algorithms do not understand or show willingness to articulate how conclusions are being derived through data analysis, this condition fails. This creates significant uncertainty about how data analysis is applied to health data now, and especially about how it could be applied in the future.

4.2.3 Persistence

Data is long-lived and duplicable; here I call the combination of these two features *persistence*. Unlike most collections of physical biological materials used for scientific and therapeutic purposes, once a collection of health data is gathered it is feasible to preserve it indefinitely and give access to it prolifically. For physical biological materials, this necessitates storage and, in cases of cell cultures, *in vitro*

[5] Here my analysis differs from Burrell's (2016) in that I do not regard widespread "technical illiteracy" about data analysis as a basic form of opacity. Ordinary people can unproblematically obtain "second-hand knowledge" from experts in many domains, even when they are technically illiterate.

reproductive techniques. For health data on a large scale, this necessitates computer storage and various means of sharing or giving access to large amounts of data.[6] Because it is quite feasible to store, copy, and access data at a "medium" scale (i.e., well below the limits of Moore's law), this leads to a potential for reproductive profligacy of health data that extends indefinitely into the future.

Persistence is a relevant source of ignorance for the data subject because many different institutions and organizations with different interests and motivations store, share, and analyze data. Vayena & Blasimme describe a "data ecosystem" with an "increasing number of stakeholders" including "the data analytics industry … [and] social media giants … [that] enter the domain of health bringing corporate cultures that are not necessarily aligned with existing regulations in health research" (2018, 121). Commercial organizations and governmental and academic institutions often cooperate in data-intensive projects, and the boundaries of data (access) are often not limited by institutional, regional, or national boundaries. Data about a person from one context or jurisdiction can be copied multiple times and shared with many different kinds of entities in different contexts or jurisdictions, with different motives (profit, surveillance, efficiency). Moreover, the results of data analysis, such as the results of profiling, become data entities of their own, which also share these features of longevity and shareability and can be distributed and reused for new purposes. In combination, these factors imply that multiple entities and types of entities (e.g., commercial entities, research entities) are likely to control one's personal health data in the long term, and that data profiles concerning data subjects are likely be generated which endure and are shared across contexts and jurisdictions.[7]

A figure (Fig. 4.1) helps to visualize this as a source of uncertainty. The lines, starting at T_0, represent the lifespan of the data. The solid lines are those parts of the lifespan under the intentional control of the original recipient or collector of data. The dashed lines represent the parts of the lifespan that are not under the intentional control of the original recipient or controller of data. These dashed lines are particularly uncertainty-inducing because they are no longer governed by the same assumptions that the data subject might have reasonably made at T_0 about the motives and interests of the entities possessing the data. The lines (both solid and dashed) can branch, of course, because parts of the data can be given away or duplicated. In addition, new branches, consisting of analyzed data or profiling data based on the original data but not identical to it, can start independently. These are represented as solid or dashed lines starting at times after T_0.

[6]Collections of biomedical samples or 'biobanks' are always associated with data, and especially where population-level biobanks are concerned this data component is just as important as the 'wet' biological component (as in the definition of the Council of Europe 2006).

[7]Deidentification of original data shared by data subjects does not prevent those subjects from being targeted in a way that resembles profiling. For example, data from patients at a particular medical practice can be deidentified and used to make generalizations about the practice, which are then used to target those very patients.

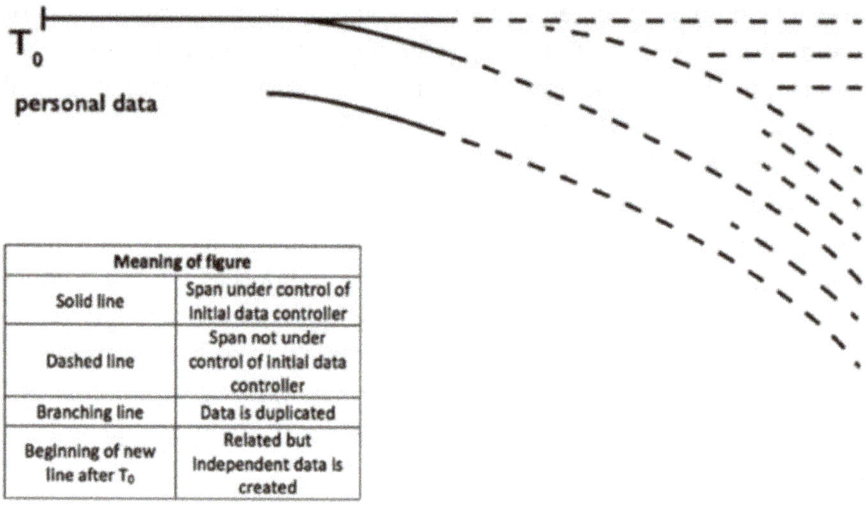

Meaning of figure	
Solid line	Span under control of initial data controller
Dashed line	Span not under control of initial data controller
Branching line	Data is duplicated
Beginning of new line after T_0	Related but independent data is created

Fig. 4.1 The persistence of personal data

4.2.4 Endemic Uncertainties Combined

The open-endedness, opacity, and persistence of data and data practices together create a host of unknowns for data subjects. Such unknowns include: how collected data about the subject will be combined in the future, how the combined data will be used to measure, classify, and profile the subject, and what implications new metrics and regimes of access to information will have for the subject. We can think of these as *unknown knowns*: they are forms of knowledge and knowledge-based power that will come into being in the future but are currently unpredictable and unknown.[8]

4.3 Two Epistemic Interests of Data Subjects

In Sect. 4.1, practical uncertainty is defined as matters that we *do not know* and have an *interest* in knowing. We have so far been focusing on those aspects of our data practices which create unknowns. Now let us turn our attention to the second part of the definition, which refers to the *interests* we have in understanding and knowing.[9]

[8] Slavoj Žižek introduced this term in relation to former U.S. Secretary of Defense Donald Rumsfeld's infamous speech about 'known unknowns' and 'unknown unknowns', in order to refer to things one does know, but does not realize or admit that they know (2004). It was later used as the title of a film about Rumsfeld by director Errol Morris. My use of the term departs from these earlier uses.

[9] Two main senses of 'interest' are operating here in a way that is mutually reinforcing: something can be *in my interest* to know, or it can be interest*ing*, or both. I use the term 'interests,' rather than

In what follows I focus on two high-priority interests that are particularly impacted by the unknowns discussed in the previous section: one's ability as a potential data subject to *trust* others with one's data, and one's ability to determine one's own *moral obligations* in relation to oneself and others where data issues are concerned. For each of these interests, I begin by presenting a case in which the relevant interest is intuitively present.

4.3.1 Interests in Trust

Shara
Shara is considering going to a hospital because she believes she may have been exposed to HIV in a sexual encounter (although she believes the risk is very low). She believes she could obtain a prescription for post-exposure HIV prophylaxis. However, she is not sure of the implications of trusting the hospital or the pharmacy with these 'data points'.

Can Shara trust the hospital and other relevant institutions with her data? Considering the uncertainties associated with institutional data practices, it might be rational for Shara to make a strategic assessment of whether the risk of HIV infection makes it worth visiting the hospital under these circumstances. She does not know who will come to possess her data in the future, how they will analyze it, and for what purposes. For all she knows, she could be profiled as being high-risk and denied service or offered different care in the future. From the perspective of individual rational choice, if not from the perspective of public health (Ford et al. 2015), such uncertainty could tip the balance in favor of not seeking treatment. This is an urgent epistemic and practical problem for Shara.

As this example illustrates, one weighty epistemic interest of data subjects is to have sufficient reason to trust entities such as governments, corporations, research institutions, and hospitals with data. Data practitioners and scholars have remarked upon this interest in trust, particularly in the health (care) domain, where trust is a bedrock value (Larson 2013; Lipworth et al. 2017). Our attitudes about the social, political, and technological world depend on trust. Trust frames how we think of our prospects for cooperation, and the responsibilities of others.

Trust involves a complex of predictive and normative expectations based on the interests, motives, and past performance of the trusted entity (Voerman and Nickel 2017). With a few notable exceptions (Hardin 2006), many scholars, including some

'rights' or 'needs,' because the latter terms presuppose that epistemic concerns are so strong as to be ethically overriding (i.e., to serve as 'trumps' over other values). I think it will be clear that the interests in question *are* sometimes sufficiently weighty to override other values or interests, but this need not always be the case.

philosophers, take for granted that one can trust institutions (Hawley 2017). We can hold this kind of trust towards specific organizations (such as Harvard University or the NHS) and various functional human roles within them (e.g., the role of data scientist or clinical researcher). Trust in institutions is based on our ideas of the norms and functional aims that govern and define organizations and the roles within them, in addition to individual characteristics such as goodwill or moral character that ground person-to-person trust (Baier 1986; Holton 1994). Trust in institutions is distinctive in that it does not normally involve the expectation that the trusted entities will be specifically responsive to the trust one places in them. In this respect, it differs from trust between intimates (Faulkner 2011).

People's interest in trust is not merely to have trust, but to have it in the right circumstances and for the right reasons. Normally, this aspect of trust is backed by having a reliable grasp of the interests, functions, and norms that motivate and explain the trusted entity's behavior. This idea of a reliable grasp can be cashed out in more 'internalist' or 'externalist' ways. Internalism means that one's warrant for trust consists primarily of items to which one has "direct and unproblematic access" (Bonjour and Sosa 2003); externalism means that it can also substantially consist of items in one's social or physical environment to which one does not have access. Manson and O'Neill (2007) put forward an ideal of 'intelligent trust' that emphasizes the virtues or talents of an individual truster in making good choices about whom to trust. Others advance a notion of 'healthy trust' or 'sound trust' that emphasizes the importance of the environment as well as the individual in creating the conditions for epistemically grounded and non-exploitative trust (Boenink 2003; Voerman and Nickel 2017). Loosely speaking, the first account emphasizes the internal aspects of warranted trust, and the second account emphasizes the external aspects. (However, the notion of "intelligent trust" could also be given an externalist interpretation, as Sosa does for the idea of intellectual virtues more generally (Bonjour and Sosa 2003).) Either way, intelligent or healthy trust depends on a stable, reliable ascription of norms and functional aims to the institutions we rely on.

The endemic uncertainties of our data practices, explicated in the previous section, threaten this epistemic basis for trust. They make it very difficult to have a stable, reliable grasp of norms and functions of the entities we rely on, or even to determine which entities are actually involved. Uncertainties about what kinds of organizations and institutions will come to possess one's data in the future, and about how data might be used for profiling, make it difficult to trust because such uncertainties threaten the warrant for trust. A data subject may reasonably wonder whether the new metrics of value-based health care might in the future be used to profile her (perhaps using an opaque algorithm) as being a poor prospect for health outcomes, or whether her data will be transferred to new entities whose motives and interests oppose her own. When such scenarios cannot be defined, the epistemic grounding for trust in health care institutions is missing. The 'what', 'how', and 'who' of trust cannot be specified.

Brown and Calnan (2012) have analyzed situations like Shara's in which there is a high degree of uncertainty and institutional complexity in clinical contexts, in terms of trust. They argue that trust becomes an explicit problem in such contexts because its rational basis is threatened (ibid., 4). However, trust remains salient as a possible way of "bridging" uncertainty (ibid., 53ff.). I follow their analysis when looking at data practices. Trust remains a possible strategy for navigating situations that arise in the midst of those practices, even when the uncertainties surrounding our data practices threaten and undermine its familiar epistemic foundation. However, such a strategy is like the Biblical house built on sand, whose foundation is unstable. It can be occupied, but existential threats to it cannot be rationally put out of one's mind.

4.3.2 Interests in Knowing Our Own Obligations

Carla
Carla has recently moved to a new area. She has a serious health problem. When she arrives at the hospital to get medical treatment for her problem, she chooses to conceal a past pregnancy and a past depression, preventing both events from becoming data points.

Is Carla failing to act in good faith? Is she unfairly advantaging herself over others in order to gain access to health care, by leaving out something that is relevant to clinical decision-making? Or is she simply protecting her privacy from exploitation by commercial and research organizations she does not endorse? Knowing one's obligations determinately means being able to answer these questions. Being morally responsible as a citizen and a member of the moral community seems to require such knowledge. Intuitively, knowing one's own obligations determinately is an important human interest.

In order to know our obligations in relation to data practices we must know who will have access to our data, what the data means for us, and how it will be used. If a patient's data will be used to profile her for unspecified purposes that extend far beyond the provision of medical care or for unrelated commercial purposes, then it seems intuitively that an act of concealment by the patient does not violate any moral duty of honesty or fairness to others but is rather a matter of protecting her own privacy. On the other hand, if the data is to be protected rigorously and used only in research that could benefit others similar to her, and her choice to conceal data actually hinders this goal, then arguably she can be seen as acting dishonestly and unfairly by not disclosing important facts from her medical history. This creates uncertainty about the duties and responsibilities conferred on different parties by a data transfer. The status of a patient's data transfer could be seen as a kind of *donation*, as the *price* of a service, or as a *shared burden*—a sort of *tax*—imposed for the sake of fairness and solidarity. Which of these ways of thinking about data transfers and their associated "deontic consequences" is the correct one is unclear and indeterminate in many cases.[10] Intuitively, this kind of moral uncertainty frustrates important interests of data subjects.

The linkage between uncertainty about our data practices and uncertainty about what obligations result from transfers of health data is implicit in Cohen's (2017) argument that people have a duty to share health data as a matter of solidarity. The argument starts with the crucial assumption that the possessor of shared health data will be either a government agency or a hospital system "committed to improving healthcare … for the people it serves," not a for-profit commercial entity (ibid., 210). When this assumption is reliably satisfied, we can think of health data sharing as having the status of a reciprocal shared burden or a tax, where everybody has an obligation to contribute, and gratitude and specific goods and services are not expected in return. Conversely, though, if there is significant uncertainty about whether data will be used for purposes unrelated to health, for commercial purposes, or by new organizations and institutions, then there will also be uncertainty about the conclusion that people have a solidaristic obligation to share health data.

An important corollary of the linkage between data practices and uncertainty is that *uncertainties about data transfers challenge the very idea of data donation*. Making a donation (i.e., gift-giving) is an act associated with other morally-laden acts and attitudes such as gratitude, and is not easy to combine with other moral regimes such as that of communitarianism and solidarity, or that of a commercial exchange (Herman 2012). In real practice, giving away data is often thought of as the *price* of using web-based services. Data is a kind of bartering chip that one uses to pay for these services. The idea of "Web 2.0" has been coined for a business model in which users are *prosumers*, who both *produce* content and data for Internet sites and applications and also *consume*—often "for free"—the valuable services that websites and apps deliver (Toffler 1980; Ritzer and Jurgenson 2010). Prosumption is a business model for many health data companies (Prainsack 2017). So long as we remain confused about whether a given data transfer is our contribution toward carrying a shared burden, as Cohen argues, or a bartering transaction, as the business model of prosumption implies, then it will not possible to consider that very transfer of data to be a pure donation at the same time.

In the remainder of this section, I address a philosophical objection to the idea that uncertainty really threatens our epistemic interests. (Those who are not worried about such an objection may choose to skip to the next section.) So far I have relied on the intuition that knowing our moral obligations determinately makes one better off. However, according to some philosophers, even if we do not know the outcomes of our actions determinately, or even the various possible ways of valuing possible outcomes, we can still calculate our moral meta-obligations (Lockhart 2000; Zimmerman 2008, 38; Barry and Tomlin 2016; Lazar 2018). The underlying strategy for determining our meta-obligations is to consider every plausible valuation of different possible actions (the possible obligations about which we are uncertain), and then use a meta-principle to calculate one's unique meta-obligation given these

[10] Compare Tutton's (2004) discussion of how to frame the "sharing" of biological materials in biobanking.

possible valuations. For example, suppose our imaginary patient Carla does not know whether her data transfer would count as a donation of data, a price that she pays in exchange for medical service, or a tax associated with the shared burden of the medical system. By taking each of these deontic statuses as members of a set of possible valuations V, she can apply a suitable meta-principle to calculate her unique actual obligation. An example of such a meta-principle might be, "If any of the valuations in V implies an obligation not to do x, then there is a meta-obligation not to do x."

This objection maintains that one's unique obligation can be specified just as well for situations of significant uncertainty as it can be for situations in which the outcomes and valuations are certain. If our knowledge of our meta-obligations under conditions of uncertainty is just as satisfactory, ethically and practically, as our knowledge of our determinate obligations, then our epistemic interest in knowing our obligations can be satisfied perfectly well even under conditions of uncertainty. This would undermine the claim that our epistemic interest in knowing our obligations is threatened by uncertainty about data practices.

This is a deep objection deserving a thorough philosophical treatment. Here I offer three preliminary replies. The first is that there is nothing that prevents us from holding that situations in which it is rational to act on a meta-principle under moral uncertainty are situations in which we are worse off, other things equal, compared to situations in which it is rational to act on a determinate principle. The second is that, empirically, people have a strong aversion to uncertainty (sometimes called "ambiguity" in the relevant empirical literature), at least in contexts where quantifiable options are directly compared to ambiguous, uncertain ones (Fox and Tversky 1995). The third is that getting the *outcome* wrong will normally be more likely if an agent does not know her own obligations determinately, than if she does. This is true even if she acts blamelessly because she acted according to an appropriate meta-principle. Being more likely to get the outcome wrong makes her worse off even if it does not reflect directly on whether she is to blame. In sum, we can accept meta-principles for situations of moral uncertainty without giving up the empirically-supported intuition that moral uncertainty threatens our interests in an important respect.

4.4 Strategies for Mitigating Uncertainty

Risk scholars have proposed structured guidelines for mitigating situations of high uncertainty, focusing on two main strategies: *increasing systemic resilience* and *reducing hazard* (Renn 2008). Since these strategies are well-established, it is useful to consider how they could be applied to the uncertainties surrounding data practices. Systemic resilience refers to *flexibility* and *organizational capacity* in monitoring and responding to ongoing hazards. Hazard reduction, by contrast, is a matter of limiting what is at stake in uncertainty. Below I attempt to identify instances of each strategy from the literature on data governance and consider whether they are likely to mitigate harms to data subjects' epistemic interests. Doing so highlights the need for further research about the feasibility of such strategies, as well as the feasibility of supplementary strategies that more directly address the problem of practical uncertainty about health data.

4.4.1 Systemic Resilience Through Flexible Systemic Oversight

First, I consider a strategy to increase systemic resilience. The General Data Protection Regulation (GDPR), taking effect in the European Union in 2018, may appear to be such a strategy. It places new governance requirements on data controllers and takes steps to harmonize governance across member countries. It requires that people be informed when they are being profiled (Regulation 2016, §60), and that people can find out the "logic involved in any personal data processing" (§63).

Despite these measures, one recent study finds that there is significant uncertainty about how the GDPR will be implemented in practice, and that there is likely to be a tradeoff between disruptive innovation and strict regulatory compliance (van den Broek and van Veenstra 2018). There are also other reasons why the GDPR does not solve the problem of uncertainty for data subjects. First, it only directly protects citizens of the EU. Second, many data subjects in the EU do not care about or understand the rights to know and to respond to data processing articulated in the GDPR, and consequently those rights do not protect them from uncertainty. Thirdly, even those who do care about their rights often give legal consent to data collection and processing because doing so is instrumental to obtaining services. Such acts of consent do not generally have the function of reducing uncertainty, as anyone who has clicked through an online consent form can ascertain.

Vayena and Blasimme (2018) have put forward the idea of flexible "systemic oversight" to avoid tradeoffs between innovation and regulatory compliance, while countering the impact of uncertainty. The idea is to create a comprehensive framework for governance that is reflexive, inclusive, and responsive. Systemic oversight is meant to allow for innovation while providing "adaptive and flexible mechanisms" for oversight, in which there is "deliberative democracy" through "collective engagement of research participants in decisions about data governance" (ibid., 124–125). In relation to uncertainty, "oversight mechanisms should not be seen as procedures for prospective risk assessment, but rather as *adaptive* instruments that respond to change" (ibid., 124).

As applied to the problems discussed here, the idea is that regulatory processes resulting from collective, democratic processes will protect data subjects' interests and thereby make the act of sharing health data more rational. Mechanisms of deliberation and collective engagement would also increase well-grounded trust (in line with the account of trust offered above in Sect. 4.3.1), so long as an alignment of interests results that favors data subjects and is available to them as a warrant for trust.

Flexible systemic oversight might be taken to mean that *relative to a given jurisdiction and use of data*, individuals could be given explicit guidance about their obligations and protected from the unexpected consequences of their choices. This could help to mitigate the effects of uncertainty about one's data-relative obligations. For example, within a given health care administrative region, the choice could be made to impose a solidaristic model of shared burden, in which everybody transfers data for the sake of common benefit. In cases where there were data leaks or unforeseen effects of profiling, a compensation scheme could be introduced to remedy the impacts, as proposed by Prainsack (2017). Such a regional choice could relieve people of the burden of uncertainty about their data-relative obligations.

Flexibility and systematicity are potentially at odds with one another, however. Flexibility implies that there is temporal and local adaptation to particular institutional situations and innovation regimes. However, this flexibility may actually prevent the formation of stable expectations that simplify trust decisions and make one's obligations as a data subject clear across different boundaries and jurisdictions. Regulation must address data that crosses the clinical/non-clinical boundary, data that crosses institutional and national borders, and data that is commercialized or exploited within public-private partnerships. Flexibility and adaptability seem to imply variability. In that case, flexible and adaptable regulatory processes may be less effective at conveying to people that their interests are being consistently protected, and less effective at establishing a simple and clear set of obligations in respect of health data, compared with truly systematic (hence inflexible) regulation with clear-cut restrictions extending to all uses and jurisdictions. More research is needed to clarify how flexibility might be balanced with systematicity, and what the impact will be on the expectations and obligations of data subjects.

4.4.2 *Hazard Reduction Through Privacy-by-Design*

Now I turn to a hazard reduction strategy. To begin with, it is important to note that it is somewhat unclear how to think about hazard reduction as applied to the data domain. In the domain of system safety, hazard reduction denotes the removal of hazardous substances and processes from a system, or their replacement with less hazardous substances and processes (Leveson et al. 2009). There is no direct analogue in the domain of privacy.

However, there are some crude parallels. We could, for example, encourage data obsolescence by default, or disallow "hypercollection" (Prainsack's (2017) term). Data obsolescence implies that after a certain time period, data is always deleted by default (it "obsolesces"), unless it has been specifically saved because of its demonstrable significance. Limiting hypercollection, by contrast, means that the default is not to collect or combine data in the first place unless there is a specific research motivation for doing so, such as a specific, powerful research question to be answered.

Although these measures could substantially protect privacy, they would carry an unacceptable cost in the health domain. They would block innovation and cost lives.

Strictly limiting data collection or encouraging data obsolescence is difficult or impossible to combine with transformative initiatives such as the value-based health care movement considered above, in which massive and persistent data collection and analysis is built into the paradigm. Obsolescence would severely limit the value of the careful work that goes into creating a dataset.

It might be possible to think of the analogue of hazard reduction strategies in the domain of privacy as a broader set of measures that limit the degree to which personal data is threatened in the first place. *Privacy-by-design* is the name applied to strategies in which privacy safeguards are built in to a technology and attended to in the primary process of technology development and implementation, incorporating physical, technical, and procedural safeguards along the way.

Understood in this way, privacy-by-design may be too broad and vague to capture the simple and obvious logic of hazard reduction, but is nonetheless promising as a strategy of mitigating uncertainty. Its effectiveness will depend upon the specifics of the situation and the way it is carried out. An important point to keep in mind is that some health data innovation appears inseparably to depend on information that can indirectly lead back to the subject (e.g., as a member of a relevant class or group) or can reidentify the subject when combined with other data (Mittelstadt et al. 2016).

4.4.3 Concluding Reflections

Health care faces major challenges such as the difficulty of efficiently caring for an aging population, and the increasing incidence of chronic diseases that are expensive to treat. Data-based innovations are one of the main ways that technology can help meet these challenges. Lives can be saved and improved by the insights gained through health data collection and analysis. At the same time, however, these innovations create many uncertainties for ordinary people. In this paper, I have argued that these uncertainties are an ethical problem for data subjects.

An important consequence for the present chapter is that in order to see a given data transfer as a *donation*, undertaken as an act of generosity, it is not possible to see it at the same time as a bartering chip that one exchanges for a service, or as a shared burden that one undertakes out of solidarity. Resolving the uncertainties around our health data may therefore mean making a choice between seeing particular data transfers in one of these ways or another. This may limit the applicability of the idea of data donation.

An important task of future research is to further develop the kinds of governance strategies discussed above so that they better address the specific epistemic problems for data donors and data subjects explored in this paper. Another is to seek complementary approaches that directly shore up trust and reduce the costs of not knowing one's own obligations.

Focusing on trust, for example, we might consider whether a greater emphasis on data *professionalism* could shore up trust in the face of uncertainty. Professionalism arises in situations where experts in some field of activity, such as doctors, engineers, and pharmacists, adopt formal standards for having the privilege of labeling themselves a certain way, and enjoy an exclusive right to evaluate the work of others who use the label. Professionalism is often linked to trust and trustworthiness (Pellegrino and Thomasma 1993; Manson and O'Neill 2007). The underlying idea is that the development of professions functions to signal trustworthiness to those with a practical need for the relevant form of expertise. Data science professionalism is relatively undeveloped compared with professionalism in other areas of science, engineering, and medicine. By developing it in the realm of health care data, and clearly signaling what standards go along with the relevant professional identity, we could create (and communicate) trustworthiness in this area.

As for our interest in knowing our own obligations in the domain of data practices, a plausible first step is for health care authorities to acknowledge openly that there is significant uncertainty about practices of data collection and analysis. This is a matter of showing respect for the real difficulties that data subjects and potential data donors face when trying to make well supported and ethically responsible decisions to accept or resist sharing data, and may be a way to begin addressing these difficulties.

Acknowledgments I would like to acknowledge the useful feedback I received on earlier versions of this paper from participants at workshops in Eindhoven, in Warwick, and at the Oxford Internet Institute. This research is affiliated with the Netherlands Organisation for Scientific Research Responsible Innovation (NWO-MVI) project "Mobile Support Systems for Behaviour Change," project number 100-23-616.

References

Altham, J.E.J. 1983. Ethics of risk. *Proceedings of the Aristotelian Society* 84: 15–29.

Baier, A. 1986. Trust and antitrust. *Ethics* 96: 231–260.

Barocas, S., and H. Nissenbaum. 2014. Big data's end run around anonymity and consent. In *Privacy, Big Data and the Public Good*, ed. J. Lane, V. Stodden, S. Bender, and H. Nissenbaum, 44–75. New York: Cambridge University Press.

Barry, C., and P. Tomlin. 2016. Moral uncertainty and permissibility: Evaluating option sets. *Canadian Journal of Philosophy* 46 (6): 898–923.

Boenink, M. 2003. Gezond vertrouwen. Over de rol van vertrouwen in het bevolkingsonderzoek naar borstkanker. *Krisis* 1: 53–74.

Bonjour, L., and E. Sosa. 2003. *Epistemic Justification: Internalism vs. Externalism, Foundations vs. Virtues*. Malden: Blackwell Publishing.

Brey, P. 2017. Ethics of emerging technology. In *The ethics of technology: Methods and approaches*, ed. S.O. Hansson, 175–191. London: Rowman & Littlefield.

Brown, P., and M. Calnan. 2012. *Trusting on the edge: Managing uncertainty and vulnerability in the midst of serious mental health problems*. Chicago: The Policy Press.

Burrell, J. 2016. How the machine 'thinks': Understanding opacity in machine learning algorithms. *Big Data and Society* 2016: 1–12. https://doi.org/10.1177/2053951715622512.

Christophersen, M., P. Mørck, T.O. Langhoff, and P. Bjørn. 2015. Unforeseen challenges: Adopting wearable health data tracking devices to reduce health insurance costs in organizations. In *International conference on universal access in human-computer interaction*, ed. M. Antona and C. Stephanidis, vol. 2, 88–99. Berlin: Springer.

Cohen, I.G. 2017. Is there a duty to share health data? In *Big data, health law, and bioethics*, ed. I.G. Cohen, H.F. Lynch, E. Vayena, and U. Gasser, 209–222. Cambridge: Cambridge University Press.

Collingridge, D. 1980. *The social control of technology*. New York: St Martin.

Committee on the Learning Health Care System in America, Institute of Medicine, Smith, M., R. Saunders, L. Stuckhardt, et al. (eds.). 2013. *Best care at lower cost: The path to continuously learning health care in America*. Washington, DC: National Academies Press. 2013 May 10. 5, A continuously learning health care system. Available from: https://www.ncbi.nlm.nih.gov/books/NBK207218/.

Council of Europe. 2006. *Recommendation Rec (2006)4 of the Committee of Ministers to Member States on Research on Biological Materials of Human Origin.*

Dereli, T., Y. Coşkun, E. Kolker, Ö. Güner, M. Ağırbaşlı, and V. Özdemir. 2014. Big data and ethics review for health systems research in LMICs: Understanding risk, uncertainty and ignorance—And catching the black swans? *The American Journal of Bioethics* 14 (2): 48–50.

Erlich, Y. 2017. Major flaws in "Identification of individuals by trait prediction using whole-genome". *bioRχiv*. https://doi.org/10.1101/185330.

Fallis, D. 2006. Epistemic value theory and social epistemology. *Episteme* 2 (3): 177–188.

Faulkner, P. 2011. *Knowledge on trust*. Oxford: Oxford University Press.

Ford, N., et al. for the World Health Organization Postexposure Prophylaxis Guideline Development Group. 2015. World Health Organization guidelines on postexposure prophylaxis for HIV: Recommendations for a public health approach. *Clinical Infectious Diseases* 60: S161–S164. https://doi.org/10.1093/cid/civ068.

Fox, C.R., and A. Tversky. 1995. Ambiguity aversion and comparative ignorance. *The Quarterly Journal of Economics* 110 (3): 585–603.

Gay, V., and P. Leijdekkers. 2015. Bringing health and fitness data together for connected health care: Mobile apps as enablers of interoperability. *Journal of Medical Internet Research* 17 (11): e260. https://doi.org/10.2196/jmir.5094.

Gillingham, P. 2016. Predictive risk modelling to prevent child maltreatment and other adverse outcomes for service users: Inside the 'black box' of machine learning. *The British Journal of Social Work* 46 (4): 1044–1058. https://doi.org/10.1093/bjsw/bcv031.

Goldberg, S. 2010. *Relying on others*. Oxford: Oxford University Press.

Goldman, A. 1999. *Knowledge in a Social World*. New York: Oxford University Press.

Hardin, R. 2006. *Trust*. Cambridge: Polity.

Hawley, K. 2017. Trustworthy groups and organizations. In *The philosophy of trust*, ed. P. Faulkner and T. Simpson, 230–250. Oxford: Oxford University Press.

Herman, B. 2012. Being helped and being grateful: Imperfect duties, the ethics of possession, and the unity of morality. *Journal of Philosophy* 109: 391–411.

Hern, A. 2014. Google: 100,000 lives a year lost through fear of data mining. *The Guardian*, June 26, 2014. https://www.theguardian.com/technology/2014/jun/26/google-healthcare-data-mining-larry-page.

Hildebrandt, M. 2009. Profiling and AmI. In *The future of identity in the information society: Challenges and opportunities*, ed. K. Rannenberg, D. Royer, and A. Deuker, 273–310. Heidelberg: Springer.

Holton, R. 1994. Deciding to trust, coming to believe. *Australasian Journal of Philosophy* 72: 63–76.

Kennedy, H., T. Poell, and J. van Dijck. 2015. Introduction: Data and agency. *Big Data and Society* 2. https://doi.org/10.1177/2053951715621569.

Knight, F. 1921. *Risk, Uncertainty, and Profit*. Boston/New York: Houghton Mifflin.

Larson, E. 2013. Building trust in the power of big data research to serve the public good. *JAMA* 309 (23): 2443–2444. https://doi.org/10.1001/jama.2013.5914.

Lazar, S. 2018. In dubious battle: Uncertainty and the ethics of killing. *Philosophical Studies* 175: 859–883.

Leveson, N., N. Dulac, K. Marais, and J. Carroll. 2009. Moving beyond normal accidents and high reliability organizations: A systems approach to safety in complex systems. *Organization Studies* 30: 227–249.

Lippert, C., et al. 2017. Identification of individuals by trait prediction using whole-genome sequencing data. *PNAS* 114 (38): 10166–10171. https://doi.org/10.1073/pnas.1711125114.

Lipworth, W., P.H. Mason, I. Kerridge, and J.P.A. Ioannidis. 2017. Ethics and epistemology in big data research. *Bioethical Inquiry* 14: 489–500.

Lockhart, T. 2000. *Moral uncertainty and its consequences*. New York: Oxford University Press.

Malin, B.A., K. El Emam, and C.M. O'Keefe. 2013. Biomedical data privacy: Problems, perspectives, and recent advances. *Journal of the American Medical Informatics Association* 20 (1): 2–6.

Manson, N., and O. O'Neill. 2007. *Rethinking informed consent in bioethics*. Cambridge: Cambridge University Press.

Mittelstadt, B.D., and L. Floridi. 2016. The ethics of big data: Current and foreseeable issues in biomedical contexts. *Science and Engineering Ethics* 22 (2): 303–341. https://doi.org/10.1007/s11948-015-9652-2.

Mittelstadt, B.D., P. Allo, M. Taddeo, S. Wachter, and L. Floridi. 2016. The ethics of algorithms: Mapping the debate. *Big Data & Society* 3 (2). https://doi.org/10.1177/2053951716679679.

Mulley, A., A. Coulter, M. Wolpert, T. Richards, and K. Abbasi. 2017. New approaches to measurement and management for high integrity health systems. *BMJ* 356: j1401. https://doi.org/10.1136/bmj.j1401.

Pellegrino, E.D., and D.C. Thomasma. 1993. *The virtues in medical practice*. New York: Oxford University Press.

Porter, M. 2009. A strategy for health care reform—Toward a value-based system. *New England Journal of Medicine* 369: 109–112.

Prainsack, B. 2017. *Personalized medicine: Empowered patients in the 21st century?* New York: NYU Press.

Regulation (EU) 2016/679 of the European Parliament and the Council. 2016. *Official Journal of the European Union*. L119/1–88.

Renn, O. 2008. White paper on risk governance: Toward an integrative approach. In *Global risk governance. International Risk Governance Council bookseries*, ed. O. Renn and K.D. Walker, vol. 1, 3–73. Dordrecht: Springer.

Rieder, G., and J. Simon. 2017. Big data: A new empiricism and its epistemic and socio-political consequences. In *Berechenbarkeit der Welt? Philosophie und Wissenschaft im Zeitalter von Big Data*, ed. W. Pietsch, J. Wernecke, and M. Ott, 85–105. Wiesbaden: Springer VS.

Ritzer, G., and N. Jurgenson. 2010. Production, consumption, prosumption. *Journal of Consumer Culture* 10: 13–36.

Sheaff, R., et al. 2015. Integration and continuity of primary care: Polyclinics and alternatives – A patient-centred analysis of how organisation constrains care co-ordination. *Health Services and Delivery Research* 3: 35. https://doi.org/10.3310/hsdr03350.

Stodden, V. 2010. *The scientific method in practice: Reproducibility in the computational sciences*, MIT Sloan School Working Paper 4773–10. Cambridge, MA: MIT Sloan School of Management.

Toffler, A. 1980. *The third wave*. New York: William Morrow.

Tutton, R. 2004. Person, property and gift: Exploring languages of tissue donation to biomedical research. In *Genetic databases: Socio-ethical issues in the collection and use of DNA*, ed. R. Tutton and O. Corrigan, 19–38. London: Routledge.

Van den Broek, T., and A.F. van Veenstra. 2018. Governance of big data collaborations: How to balance regulatory compliance and disruptive innovation. *Technological Forecasting and Social Change* 129: 330–338.

Vayena, E., and A. Blasimme. 2018. Health research with big data: Time for systemic oversight. *The Journal of Law, Medicine & Ethics* 46: 119–129.

Voerman, S.A., and P.J. Nickel. 2017. Sound trust and the ethics of telecare. *Journal of Medicine and Philosophy* 42: 33–49.

Wang, Y., and M. Kosinski. 2018. Deep neural networks are more accurate than humans at detecting sexual orientation from facial images. *Journal of Personality and Social Psychology* 114 (2): 246–257.

Wynne, B. 1992. Uncertainty and environmental learning. *Global Environmental Change* 2: 111–127.

Zimmerman, M.J. 2008. *Living with uncertainty: The moral significance of ignorance*. Cambridge: Cambridge University Press.

Žižek, Slavoj. 2004. What Rumsfeld doesn't know that he knows about Abu Ghraib. *These Times*. Accessed on 4 March 2018 at http://www.lacan.com/zizekrumsfeld.htm.

Chapter 5
Incongruities and Dilemmas in Data Donation: Juggling Our 1s and 0s

Kerina H. Jones

Abstract The creation of vast, complex datasets made possible by technological advances over recent decades, has resulted in data becoming big business across many sectors and disciplines world-wide. Everyday life is increasingly networked via a growing array of digital devices to which individuals provide data, passively and actively. The pace of development has led to questions about the role of such 'data donors' and how individuals can be safeguarded when they might not be fully cognisant of the extent or destinations of data provided. We show that the many ways in which individuals provide data about themselves can result in incongruities and dilemmas in apparent decision making. We argue that it is not ethical for the vast swathes of data provided by individuals not to be used for public good. We explore whether we can make truly informed choices with the panoply of issues that may influence our decisions. We conclude without a straightforward yes or no, but propose that if we provide the best available information and engage with information presented, we stand a more reasonable chance. Do that, there is a need for demonstrable trustworthiness and clarity, greater awareness so that trust can be placed wisely, and for us to hone our juggling skills.

Keywords Data donation · Incongruities · Dilemmas · Big data · Tissue/organ donation

5.1 Introduction

The etymology of the word 'donation' is from the latin 'donum' meaning 'gift', with the French 'donner', to give, being a familiar derivative. It has been proposed that it can be easier to donate blood and even organs than to donate our data. This appears incongruous, and raises questions about the contexts and rationales for these positions. Using the donation of general personal data and health data in

K. H. Jones (✉)
Population Data Science, Swansea University Medical School, Swansea, UK
e-mail: k.h.jones@swansea.ac.uk

J. Krutzinna, L. Floridi (eds.), *The Ethics of Medical Data Donation*,
Philosophical Studies Series 137, https://doi.org/10.1007/978-3-030-04363-6_5

example scenarios, this discursive chapter explores areas such as: alternative consent models; the unknown element in data content; trust and trustworthiness in data custodians; and meaningful public engagement, to consider the bioethical balance between individual autonomy, personal exploitation and social responsibility. Ultimately, the question is whether we, as individuals and society, can make truly informed choices with the panoply of issues that may influence our decisions, creating dilemmas as we juggle our 1s and 0s.

5.2 Hast Thou Which Art but *Data*, a Touch, a Feeling?[1]

Digital data at the most fundamental level is represented as a combination of 1s and 0s. Over recent decades, major technological advances have enabled the creation of vast, complex datasets commonly referred to as 'big data'. Big data is big business: it has been estimated that its worth to the UK will exceed £320 billion by 2020, and that in the US, the m-health app market alone will reach almost $60 billion in the same timescale (Greenbaum 2018; City a.m. 2017). There is a global profusion of enterprises seeking to make the best use of person-based data to inform policy, health and other public services, business, marketing and an array of other commercial and non-commercial developments for public good and/or profit. There has never been such a high demand for our personal data to be donated, such that it is often said that individuals are the product, not just the client (Wu 2017). But before we begin considering data donation, it's worth highlighting that data ownership is a tricky concept in law. It's something we often refer to informally e.g. my data, your data, but laws of ownership mainly relate to people owning tangible items, such as objects or property, and data does not fit neatly into these categories. The question arises as to how someone can be said to own data, since in order to be meaningful, ownership should confer a concept of possession. Furthermore, tangible items are generally exhaustible whereas data are not, but can be used repeatedly by multiple parties for multiple purposes *ad infinitum*. With this in mind, it is indeed difficult to see how someone can be said to own their data since once the data are known to others, the person no longer has real control over their fate.

Rather than ownership, data protection legislation and regulations relate to safeguarding the privacy of data subjects and the confidentiality of the information in question. Within the EU, we have seen the recent introduction of the General Data Protection Regulation (GDPR, EU GDPR portal 2018), with concomitant national legislation, marking an overhaul in the way personal data are governed. The GDPR enhances the rights of individuals as data subjects, and it places a greater onus on data controllers and processors to justify proactively their lawful basis for using personal data, including providing suitable privacy notices for data subjects. But it doesn't ultimately change the fundamental focus on data protection rather than data ownership.

[1] Hast thou, which art but air, a touch, a feeling. (Shakespeare, The Tempest).

Article 4 (1) of the GDPR (Intersoft consulting 2017) defines personal data as: *'any information relating to an identified or identifiable natural person'*, and *'an identifiable natural person'* as *'one who can be identified, directly or indirectly, in particular by reference to an identifier such as a name, an identification number, location data, an online identifier or to one or more factors specific to the physical, physiological, genetic, mental, economic, cultural or social identity of that natural person'*. Article 6 (1) sets out the six lawful bases for general data processing, and Article 9 sets the provisions for processing special category data, which is defined as: *'personal data revealing racial or ethnic origin, political opinions, religious or philosophical beliefs, or trade union membership, and the processing of genetic data, biometric data for the purpose of uniquely identifying a natural person, data concerning health or data concerning a natural person's sex life or sexual orientation '* (Intersoft consulting 2017). Even so, it can be argued that we haven't yet uncovered all the types of data that could be seen as personal, and which could yet necessitate a further update in legislation. We are seeing a rapid increase in connectedness via urban monitoring, the internet of things and smart objects, some within our own homes or even as our clothing (Engineering & Technology 2017). Interestingly, the Article 29 Working Party on Data Protection already broadens the scope of health data, accepting that lifestyle data may constitute health data if they are inherently related to a person's health status (Article 29 Data Protection Working Party 2013). We engage in in-depth (sometimes rather personal) conversations on social media, accept store loyalty cards which track our purchases, and use a variety of lifestyle apps on our devices. The genomic revolution is opening up untold opportunities for research and medicine, that were not available just a few years ago. There is a myriad of occasions where we donate our data, either actively or passively, as we go about our daily business or take part in dedicated activities. Altogether we are creating a rich data footprint, sometimes without knowing which types of data have been collected, by whom, or even having no awareness of them at all.

5.3 What We Might Be Donating

For the purpose of this chapter, we will stick with the concept of donation as gifting something to another party or parties, even though it is not as straightforward in the donation of data as it is for more tangible objects. Our data subject, let's call him Schrödinger's Pat[2], might passively or actively donate personal data from many sources to various parties, over the course of his life or after his death. This may include data from his: health and administrative records, DNA, social media posts, mobile phone call detail records, apps, and store loyalty cards. He might also donate blood, stem cells, tissue samples and paired organs during his life, then vital organs

[2] Schrödinger's cat: a quantum physics thought experiment where a cat may be simultaneously alive and dead.

or his whole body after his death. Importantly to remember is that whatever is donated, data are being generated.

Pat might donate general and special category data to different parties for different purposes, with or without his full awareness. It can be easy, possibly too easy, to donate data in some instances. For example, we readily sign up for store loyalty cards on the promise of discounts or rewards, but it is important to remember that the data collected as we shop is of more value to the store than any benefits to the customer. Similarly with social media platforms; we gain the benefits of social contact, but our data may be used to target us for marketing and sometimes for other reasons. The recent Facebook debacle over psychological profiling by Cambridge Analytica is a case in point, where it has been alleged that personal data from a personality quiz on Facebook was used to try and manipulate voting intentions. People engaging in the quiz were unwittingly providing detailed information about themselves to be used for illicit purposes (Solon and Graham-Harrison 2018).

Pat might also choose to use health or fitness apps which collect special category data, such as diagnoses, medications and medical symptoms. Or he may choose to engage with a Direct to Consumer (DTC) DNA sequencing company to find out about his genetic susceptibility to certain conditions. DTCs provide information to customers for a fee, but generally use the data for business development, research and to sell to third parties in anonymised or aggregated form. Questions have been raised about the rectitude of DTC services, since individuals might be ill-equipped to deal with the results, and the actual predictive value of the information provided might not live up to company marketing promises (Cussins 2018). Some countries have banned DTCs and others are considering their legislation in this regard (Kalokairinou et al. 2017).

As well as donating data (in the form of data) Pat might donate blood, tissue or organs during the course of his life, or after his death. This, of course, also generates data. Within Wales, and soon to be implemented in England, there is an opt-out consent mechanism whereby a person donates their organs after death, unless they had previously opted out. It is an interesting incongruity that we have an opt out system for organ donation after death, but we do not have a similar arrangement in place for data donation after death. Yet, organs can be used to generate rich data, including full genome sequences of living relatives of the deceased, and thus may uncover highly-sensitive familial information compared to health record data that, paradoxically, cannot be shared in this way. However, it could be argued that it is the opt out consent system for posthumous organ donation that is ethically at fault, since a forced or presumed gift loses the spirit of being a gift (McCartney 2017). The question arises as to whether we can be sure the public genuinely feel they were informed about the process, or if a significant proportion just haven't engaged, and simple inertia has prevented them from going on-line to opt out. We will explore this concept in more detail.

5.4 Are We at Least with Socrates?

Whether or not Socrates actually said he was the wisest man because he was aware he knew nothing, it is an apt sentiment in gauging our own perspectives, and one we can apply in relation to data donation. For the many ways in which Pat might donate data in one form or another, the level to which he is informed and the nature of consent may vary widely. Medical research is generally well-regulated but, across other domains, Pat may give his permission to donate data via everything from properly informed consent to 'agreeing' to lengthy terms & conditions. This is a common problem and one for which there has been a number of social experiments. In a survey completed by 550 DTC customers, most respondents considered themselves aware of privacy issues, and the risk of troubling repercussions of data donation to be negligible. But over 50% men and almost 30% women also said they had not read the terms & conditions (Haeusermann et al. 2017). Among a group of over 500 students signing up to a fictitious social media channel, none of them read the terms & conditions well enough to notice that they had agreed to hand over their first-born child (Technica UK 2016). These studies warrant an exclamation mark(!) and leave us in doubt about the adequacy of consent processes in some spheres. They highlight the dilemma of where the responsibility lies in engaging properly with the public, as to whether the onus should be more on the individual or the data collector. In answer to our own Socratic question, it appears that no, we often don't know that we don't know.

5.5 Legal Position – Data vs Tissue

The EU GDPR, and related new national legislation, might be the hero to save us from some of these difficulties. Under the GDPR, the requirements for valid informed consent have been tightened, such that Recital 32 states that *'consent should be given by a clear affirmative act establishing a freely given, specific, informed and unambiguous indication of the data subject's agreement to the processing of personal data relating to him or her'* (Intersoft consulting 2017). This places new limits on the use of opt-out consent mechanisms and on the use of lengthy, tiny wordy, scrolly downy, nobody readsy, terms & conditions. This move, together with the requirement for greater clarity on data processing in privacy notices, the right of individuals to request a copy of data pertaining to them, and the right of data erasure, serves to empower individuals on the use of their personal data. As soon as the GDPR came into force, complaints were brought against Facebook, Google and others, alleging that companies are forcing users to accept targeted advertising, or to delete their accounts (Foxx 2018). If these complaints are upheld, and as more users become aware of their rights, this could result in serious financial and reputational damage for these companies. Hopefully, it will bring about a change in practice to respect data donors and comply properly with the regulations. Other social media giants, notably Twitter, have introduced clear, granular controls that allow users more choice, including opting out of targeted advertising which relies on user profiling (Foxx 2018).

We have already mentioned posthumous organ donation, but there is also tissue and organ donation from living individuals to consider, with the corresponding implications for the individuals and their kin. The UK, in common with many countries, has specific legislation governing the donation of human tissue from living individuals (UK Human Tissue Act 2004). Organisations processing human tissue must be licensed, abide by strict protocols and are subject to inspections by regulatory authorities. However, with the advancing genomic revolution, tissue donated by one consented individual can generate increasingly rich information about the donor and their kin, as the secrets of DNA are being uncovered. Yet, it would not be practicable or ethical to seek consent from all the possibly relevant individuals. For *bone fide* organisations we rely on good governance regimes for data management and access; but with the explosion of interest in genomic data, and huge multinational companies such as Apple, Google and Amazon entering the health market, it is not known what the future holds or whether the ensuing power-play will yet trump bioethical factors one way or another (Scott 2018).

5.6 No Man Is an Island Entire of Itself[3]

When Pat chooses whether to donate any kind of personal data about himself, he needs to remember that his decision will have implications for others. On the basis of Western philosophy, we lean on the side of individual autonomy in our bioethical principles. The four main principles we commonly rely on being: (i) the rights of individuals to make decisions and to be provided with truthful, complete information to be able to make a properly informed choice, free from coercion (autonomy); (ii) not intentionally harming individuals through acts of commission or omission, and providing standards of care meeting the law and commonly held moral convictions (non-maleficence); (iii) a duty to benefit individuals, and actively preventing harm (beneficence); and (iv) equality and fairness in the provision of care and distribution of resources by seeking to overcome disadvantages (justice) (Beauchamp and Childress 2013). But, if we are to give due consideration to data donation, individuals also have to face the concept of social responsibility, with the added dilemma of whether in the act of donating we are potentially benefitting or harming others associated with us. This can be the case in many contexts, and it not limited to the obvious genomic data example. It has been observed that some apps used on social media platforms seek access to the user's contact list and photographs, and it is worth carefully reviewing privacy settings to be sure we are aware of the data donation 'choices' we are making (Denholm 2016).

[3] No man is an island (John Donne).

Although we have referred to bioethical principles, it is interesting to consider the extent to which our data donation decisions are based on bioethics or on other considerations altogether. When we donate personal data to a research project having a defined protocol, clear aims and anticipated outcomes, with potential risks and benefits for participants, we could reasonably say we choose our position based on our moral perspectives. We might hope for benefits for ourselves, or we might be acting altruistically in undergoing an intrusive process purely for the future benefit of others, based on a sense of social responsibility. But when we donate data in other contexts, such as social media, it is doubtful that we base our decisions on ethics. Similarly with choosing to use an app, a DTC company, or a mobile phone contract. A key difference seems to be in the purpose of the transaction. Participating in a research project carries the concept of 'giving something back' and thus contributing to the good of society. Signing up to use a service or product, however, is rather different, as it is directly associated with obtaining something based on need or desire. As we've observed, we are often presented with a potentially coercive situation where we can only obtain the item if we enter into the agreement. Ironically, we are often taken stepwise through a process to donate data to research for public good, with much less attention paid as we rush to complete the transaction to gain the prize in the latter scenarios. Furthermore, the extent to which the companies with whom we engage are acting on the four ethical principles might be highly variable when profit is their primary purpose. In some cases, this might be more akin to personal exploitation by platforms of largely unaccountable power.

5.7 Data, Data Everywhere, nor any Chance to Think[4]

So if it's only partly about bioethics, it will be valuable to consider what else shapes Pat's choices and the norms of society concerning data donation. We have noted that data might be provided passively or actively and in multiple contexts as we go about our daily lives. In general, we are all subject to vast amounts of potentially influential information from many sources. Unlike in the past, our challenge is not in finding information, but in knowing how to be judicious in selecting what is reliable enough to guide our decisions. Depending how we view the commonly-referred to 'information society', we might see ourselves as the most privileged generation yet, or the one most subject to the attention merchants (Wu 2017). Estimates vary, but reviews indicate that about 2.5 million academic articles are published every year, challenging professionals to keep abreast of cutting edge knowledge to inform their practice (Ware and Mabe 2015). As members of the public with our respective areas of expertise and ignorance, we are bombarded with information on any number of topics from multiple angles and media outlets. It is difficult to ignore information once it is known to us: it is assessed for its value or resides in our subconscious

[4] Water, water everywhere, nor any drop to drink (The Rime of the Ancient Mariner, Samuel Taylor Coleridge).

waiting to become relevant. Altogether, we are subject to a vast, shifting body of knowledge that floats around shaping our social realities.

We might sometimes be relatively disengaged, and perhaps we need to be, from much of the information that comes our way. If we were to ask people travelling on a train, or in another common social setting, whether they have donated any data today, we are likely to receive puzzled looks or responses in the negative. Yet, unless we are disconnected from the digital realm, it is highly unlikely that we have not donated data in some form to someone over the course of a day. But, at times, we may find ourselves in a position where we need to make important decisions about data donation. It is on these days where we hit the personal threshold, that our worldview and bioethical principles come to the fore, and we find ourselves needing to draw upon the information available to us to navigate a moral maze. This might relate to decisions about our own (or a loved one's) health, finances, education or any of an array of issues that may impact on our personal lives, taking us beyond our public personas and into the domain we consider private. At times like this, we are likely to become more concerned that we can trust the recipients of our data and their motives, as we have to move out of our, sometimes, blasé bubbles. But by this time, we are already likely to have a substantial data footprint, which may not have been donated so thoughtfully. Perhaps it is time to re-evaluate.

5.8 Up in the Air

All things considered, we propose that there are indeed incongruities in data donation, and that we find ourselves juggling our 1s and 0s between different parties and purposes. Taking Pat as our data subject, he might donate different types of data via the same basic decision-making process, or the same data via very different processes. For example, if he uses a variety of apps, he is able to donate general personal data such as his location via a fitness monitoring app, or his medical data via a health-monitoring app reminding him when to take his medication or recording self-reported symptoms to monitor a chronic condition. Alternatively, and more starkly, he might donate health (including genomic) data to a company by remote agreement to terms & conditions via a web-based agreement form. Or he might donate the very same data to a medical researcher as part of a clinical trial, via one-to-one consultation carried out on a face-to-face basis. As mentioned above, the legitimacy of DTC companies is in question in some domains (Kalokairinou et al. 2017), but perhaps we should also be more cognisant about health-monitoring apps that are not controlled solely by our care provider, but are run by third parties primarily for gain arising from the data harvested. It is possible that when our decisions are made remotely, in the 'privacy' of our own homes, our attention is cocooned by the sense of security created by our familiar environment. But of course, this is irrelevant for digitally-connected transactions even if we may feel 'safe' when signing up on our own device. In some scenarios, Pat could be in the position of not knowing the recipients of his data, exactly what data items have been collected, or what will be done with them by whom. The original recipient may further process the data and pass it on, or sell it, to other parties albeit in anonymised format.

5.9 Through a Glass Darkly[5]

In these respects, it can be too easy to donate personal data, as even if data have been through a process of anonymisation, it might not be impossible to derive some identifiable information from within them by attribution. This is commonly referred to as 'jigsaw' or 'mosaic' attack and in some cases can lead re-identification (UK Anonymisation Network 2018). Many studies have shown that the removal of commonly recognised identifiers (such as name and address) is insufficient to render a dataset truly anonymous. This is because of residual risks due to the presence of unique records. As a possibly surprising example, 87% of people in the US have been shown to have a unique combination of birth date, sex and zip code. Such information provides a fast-track to uncovering individual identity and has led some authors to lament the broken promises of anonymisation (Ohm 2010). Uncovering individual identity is a sufficient problem in itself, but it doesn't stop there. By using information from public sources and anonymised health data, it has been shown that the confidential health records of specific individuals can be uncovered. Famously, this occurred to a Governor of Massachusetts, where a researcher deduced and sent his health records to his office with 'theatrical flourish' (Ohm 2010)! This problem further extends to genomic data, with its implications for kin as well as for the data donor. Researchers used an open-access genetic database detailing short tandem repeats on the Y-chromosome, and used genetic similarity to infer familiality in the paternal line. By combining these similarities with information on a publically-accessible genealogy database containing surnames, they were able to reveal cases where recorded paternity and genetics did not correspond. This could obviously have serious implications for the personal lives and familial relationships of the data donors (Gymrek et al. 2013). Clearly, there needs to be something more than purported anonymisation if Pat's privacy is to be secured.

All is certainly not lost as there are many *bone fide* enterprises across the world where privacy-by-design is an integral concept with a strong emphasis on good data governance[6]. Privacy-by-design is an important whole system concept where a suite of controls is built in at all stages in working with person-based data (Intersoft consulting 2017). The environment surrounding the data is designed to be conducive to safe data storage and use, providing stronger data governance regimes than relying

[5] 1 Corinthians 13:12 (The Holy Bible).

[6] International examples – Secure Anonymised Information Linkage Databank https://saildatabank.com/; Institute for Clinical and Evaluative Sciences https://www.ices.on.ca/; Population Data BC https://www.popdata.bc.ca/; Population Health Research Network http://www.phrn.org.au/; and Scottish Informatics and Linkage Collaboration http://www.datalinkagescotland.co.uk/

on data curtailment alone. It can be a challenge to strike the optimum balance between data privacy and utility, as controls applied to datasets to limit the risk of disclosure may compromise research utility. Some examples could be aggregating age into 10-year bands, or suppressing outlying variables, depending on the research question of interest. It can be easy to be drawn into what has been termed 'privacy perfectionism', where superfluous controls are applied to datasets diminishing data utility but without providing additional safeguards (Allen et al. 2013). This is where privacy-by-design comes in as it combines physical, technical and procedural controls to provide more robust and flexible data protection (Jones et al. 2014; Pencarrick Hertzman et al. 2013).

As well as addressing the safe use of health data in general, there is considerable debate in the literature over whether genetic data need to be treated as a special case for data protection. This has been termed 'genetic exceptionalism' (Chin and Campbell 2013). As a concept, it flies in the face of some current initiatives, which aim to make genetic data open and publically-accessible. This is the established pattern with platforms for genome referencing and genome-wide association studies (GWAS) (GeneCards 2018), but more recently, there are initiatives where genetic data together with general health data (sometimes plus demographics) are being shared openly. An example of this is the Personal Genome Project (PGP) (Personal Genome Project 2018) where individuals engaging with the project can choose to make their linked health and genetic data publically accessible via a website. The PGP is clear in the information it provides to participants, including the possible risks to their privacy, such that individuals engage with their eyes open (providing they read the information properly!). Sharing data in this way can be seen as an impressive altruistic gesture, but it does also raise risks for the individual and their kin, as we have alluded to earlier. Relatives of a data donor may unwittingly be exposed to others knowing their estimated likelihood of developing a genetic condition, or of the information falling into the hands of parties who might use it to deny them employment or insurance. It is noteworthy that the GDPR does not especially single out genetic data, but classifies them along with general health data under Article 9 (Intersoft consulting 2017). Research has shown that among the general public there is almost an even split among those who think genetic data is different to other health data and those that either do not, or who are unsure (52% yes; 48% no/unsure) (Global Alliance for Genomics and Health 2017). The bioethical debate continues and is likely to do so for some time with new revelations being made about the genome. Without wishing to raise concerns unnecessarily, as individuals considering our options in donating data, we need to move away from the naïve concept that data are anonymised just because we are told this is the case. Again we come back to the judicious use of information from the plethora available to us, and the challenges this presents.

5.10 Life Through a Lens (Or Several)

By the time the information on which we base our data donation choices reaches us, it is likely to have passed through a number of filters affecting its interpretation and presentation to us, as well as to decision makers who may be acting on our behalf. Concepts can be magnified, diminished or fragmented as information passes via a series of intermediaries, with their interpretations acting as lenses, variously refracting the information and influencing the next steps. A decision maker has to be judicious in use of the information available in making choices affecting the use of their, or another's data, but information provenance might not be fully known.

This is a universal problem, not limited to the information sources already considered. Importantly, this also highlights challenges in the interpretation and implementation of privacy legislation and information governance frameworks, which may influence our decisions, and those who provide us with guidance. In a review of harms arising from the use of health and biomedical data, it was shown that the most prevalent cause of data misuse was the maladministration of data governance, rather than wilful data abuse (Laurie et al. 2015; Stevens et al. 2017). This included failures to follow correct procedures, despite guidance and the existence of standard procedures and protocols, and failures to take action to avoid data misuse taking place. The report included recommendations for improved staff training amongst other measures to strengthen information governance practice (Laurie et al. 2015; Stevens et al. 2017). However, as well as protecting proper individual privacy and safeguarding professionals, it can sometimes be the case that rules are over-stringent or their true essence is lost in translation.

The review also covered harm due to the non-use of health data. This is seen as a distinct issue and not merely the reverse of gaining the benefits of data used properly. This aspect of the work showed that there are instances where poor information governance can result in serious repercussions for individuals and society. Some pertinent causes of this problem were: lengthy and duplicative approval processes, conflicting advice, and excessive disclosure controls applied to de-identified data, limiting its utility. The apparent reasons were often quite straightforward but problematic nonetheless. They included: unclear lines of responsibility, fear of making the wrong decisions, and alterations to organisational data governance frameworks in the absence of legislative or regulatory changes. As a result, there can be a skew or deficit in the information available to data donors, like Pat, and the professionals who provide his care (Jones et al. 2017). We will return to the issue of data non-use later in this chapter. As a general rule whether we're acting as individuals or professionals, we should always seek the most definitive information, as close to the primary source as possible, when we make decisions on donating data. But, of course, we may not know the derivation of the information that reaches us, and this may leave us with a dilemma we can't really quantify, whilst needing to proceed one way or the other.

5.11 Minding Our Ps and Qs

So, with all this in mind, let's look at what we can do to raise realistic awareness. One major action is to stop asking questions that cannot be answered. In engaging with the public, there is little point in simply asking whether people think their personal data should be used or not. Sometimes data have to be used for various essential purposes, and at other times data are being used with negligible regard for social acceptability. Public engagement researchers have mostly moved on to asking more focused and answerable questions, such as how data should be used and by whom. In seeking to make public engagement meaningful, there is a need to be upfront about what we know and what we do not know. Keeping with tradition, we can use some alliteration in elaborating this point. These are at least some of the unknown Ps we need to grapple with: the package (the data content); the parties (the data users); the purpose (the data uses); and the places (the data environment).

Unless Pat obtains a copy, he would not be alone in not knowing the full details of data held about him by a given data controller. As an aside, with the introduction of the GDPR, he is now in a position where he may request this is if he wishes to do so (Intersoft consulting 2017). Two key areas where the unknown package is likely to be most pronounced, but for different reasons, are on major social media, search and retail platforms and in genomic data. It is well-known that companies such as Facebook, Google and Amazon use advanced data-scraping algorithms to source as much online information as possible about their users. This puts Pat in a position, whether he's aware of it or not, that he really doesn't know the scope or extent of data held about him and his online activities. On the contrary, with genomic data, it is the full meaning of the dataset itself that is unknown. Even with a copy of the data, Pat would not know what it all means, since that knowledge is just not available. In these scenarios, when we donate data we do so without fully knowing what they contain.

When the public are asked, they generally express differing levels of willingness to donate data to different parties. Unsurprisingly, the trend is usually in favour of non-commercial organisations and less so for the commercial sector. This is true for general health data, administrative data arising from other public services and, unsurprisingly, for genomic data (Global Alliance for Genomics and Health 2017; Cameron et al. 2014; Ipsos MORI 2016). But across all sectors, we might not have full knowledge of the parties themselves or others to whom they may pass the data; and in the act of giving the matter more thought we might even skew our own perspectives. The extent to which this may occur depends on many factors, including the body of information that shapes our personal views and the most pervasive current events in the media. It can be easy to demonise certain sectors wholescale, disregarding that they are not all one entity. This can be seen in public views on the pharmaceutical industry, towards whom distrust is often expressed. Although there have been some high-profile cases where pharma companies have behaved inappropriately with data (Cohen 2014; Goldacre 2013), poor research integrity is not necessarily limited to the private sector. It's also worth remembering that pharma companies create the majority of our medicines, and the cost of bringing a new drug to market can stretch to $billions (Herper 2017). This requires a major commitment and is one unlikely to be embarked on frivolously; although they profit, they also produce public good. When we engage with the public, or we are the individuals being engaged with, we need to take broader issues into account, beyond the immediate. For example, by remembering that we donate our data to other major organisations, such as via social media, with far less consideration and knowledge than participating in a research study, whether commercial or non-commercial. In this way, we can hope to gain a fuller picture before we make our decisions.

This leads nicely to the purposes for which our donated data are used, of which there will be far too many to consider here. But we can take a basic division between primarily for-profit and not-for-profit. Again, we are likely to be more permissive towards not-for-profit uses of our data. But even so, it is sometimes difficult to know exactly how data will be used. This is less likely to be an issue with data we provide as part of our receipt of healthcare. However, this is not failsafe, as there have been rare cases where large volumes of National Health Service data have been passed to third parties without due governance and leading to an outcry in the media (Hern 2017). Properly-governed research from any sector should ideally include a research protocol with defined questions and data requirements. Clinical trials of medicinal products tend to have tightly-controlled specifications from the outset. But in other research designs, it is not always desirable or even possible to be completely definitive at the start. Often research studies need to build in a degree of flexibility whilst operating within the bounds of regulatory approvals, including having a relevant lawful basis for processing the donated data. Where participant consent is relied upon, it must be properly informed and freely given. Thus we may have a conundrum in some research scenarios: unknown elements vs the need to inform. When this occurs, it is the duty of researchers to be upfront in the recruitment process so that participants have the best information available on which to base their decisions. Across other for-profit domains where Pat may donate his data, the purposes of data use could be vaguer and more exploitative, as we've noted earlier.

As well as a measure of unknowns in the package, parties and purposes, we may also be faced with uncertainties in the places: that is, in the data environment. Data could be stored and managed in a myriad of ways, just some of which are outlined briefly since this is a vast subject beyond the scope of this chapter. They might reside in anything from a simple, locally-held database under the control of a single individual to a large-scale platform with privacy-by-design. The data could be stored on a single PC, on a local server, or on a cloud-based storage system operating across jurisdictions. They could be publically accessible, or subject to access restrictions, and they could be released externally or retained within a data safe haven. How and where the data are to be held is an essential data governance issue for the safe, secure use of data. It calls for assurance that security measures have been applied to mitigate risks, and that the data custodians can be considered trustworthy. This is needful, not just to satisfy regulatory authorities, but also in communicating with, and respecting, individuals donating their data. It is part of conveying transparent information to promote informed choice. Of course, it might not be appropriate to describe the security model and control measures in technical detail, but it is important to do so in a way that enables individuals to understand the principles of how their data will be handled and protected. Again, it's about clarity and the limits thereof. To complete our consideration of Ps and Qs, we ask what we can best do, and we propose that: as professionals we should be honest about uncertainty to the best of our knowledge; and as individuals, we should recognise that there are sometimes limits in knowledge when working with data. Even so, all must be conducted with integrity and trustworthiness on all sides.

5.12 The Need for Innovation in Data Governance

Having established some of the many complexities and uncertainties to be taken into account in data donation, we propose that there is a strong need for innovation in data governance so that the best use of data can be made in safe, socially-acceptable ways. Pat's data are subject to a range of factors influencing their transformation into information, not limited to the specifications of legislation and regulations. There is a complex interplay between legislation and regulations, how they are interpreted and the body of knowledge that influences this process, such that the realisation of information from Pat's data, in all its manifestations, is dependent on a variety of factors. These instruments give rise to broader ethical, legal and societal issues (ELSI), implementation frameworks and due diligence processes. In line with the famous adage that 'in theory there is no difference between theory and practice: in practice there is', implementation is dependent on interpretation. Different individuals and organisations will have their own perceptions, risk appetites and motivations in coming to an opinion on a data governance issue. As well as that, these perceptions are coloured by the body of opinion coming from stakeholders and the wider media. In these respects, this is a prime example of our life through a lens illustration. As we've noted, the 'big data' landscape is one that is expanding rapidly, with increases not just in data volumes but also in data types being donated. These emerging types, such as genomic, imaging, free-text, social media and smart object data can stretch current data governance regimes. They call for innovative solutions to avoid undue bureaucracy and support the safe, socially-acceptable use of donated data. It is a positive step that the GDPR has introduced measures to strengthen individual rights over their personal data, and to limit exploitative activities such as automated profiling (Intersoft consulting 2017). But even so, data analytics often run in advance of ELSI-based solutions, particularly in areas where data are seen as a lucrative commodity. Thus, there is a need for innovation to enable safe, effective data use without undue bureaucracy.

5.13 Who Are You, Who, Who, Who, Who?[7]

By now, we might really want to know what our role as individuals and professionals can be or should be in relation to the complex issue of data donation. This, of course, will depend on a multiplicity of factors, and is really only a question we can answer for ourselves in relation to each data donation instance. But it is worth considering some of the factors that may dictate our role. Firstly, our views are likely to be strongly influenced depending whether we ourselves are the data donor, whether they relate to our close kin, and the perceived sensitivity of the likely data content. Whether we realise it fully or not, our thinking is shaped by our worldview and the vast, shifting body of knowledge that floats around shaping our social realities that we mentioned earlier. We also have the urgency of the issue versus the distance from the issue, and whatever defines that concept in a given instance. Furthermore, as we have shown, we are often likely to be dealing with incomplete information on which to base our choices. Altogether, it's not surprising that Pat may find himself in a quandary when he has to come out of his comfort zone and make important decisions about his data. Though painful, this can actually be a good thing, on the basis that at least he can question his position and the information being presented to him in making his choices. For Pat, and any of us, there are likely to be occasions where we need to take on different roles to fulfil our familial and social responsibilities. We might be leading, shaping a situation, or basically a follower guided by others. The key, in all cases is to seek and provide the best available information to inform decisions. There are various versions of the phrase: 'without data, all decisions are guesswork', and ultimately, our aim is the safe, socially-acceptable, increasing use of data for public good. The alternative is unthinkable.

5.14 Finding the Black Cat in the Dark Room

There is no doubt that data saves lives, and this phrase itself is the rallying cry of a major public engagement campaign to highlight the value of health data, and to encourage people to pledge their support for their safe re-use in research for the benefit of individuals and society (Farr Institute of Health Informatics Research 2018). Earlier, we looked briefly at the influence of poor information governance practice on the non-use of health data. Let's look at the implications of data non-use in a little more detail. The aforementioned international case study covered the non-use of health data across clinical records and research domains, as well as in relation to governance regimes (Jones et al. 2017). From this study, it became evident that there are multiple reasons for data non-use, compounding each other and resulting in serious harm to individuals and society. As a result, health data non-use has been strongly implicated in hundreds of thousands of deaths and £billions in financial

[7] Who are you? (Pete Townsend, The Who).

burdens to societies (Jones et al. 2017). It is a challenging issue to study, as harm due to data non-use is difficult to attribute unequivocally, but there is no doubt that this black cat certainly is there. The study concluded that, although there are many initiatives seeking to address this problem, much more needs to be done. The most effective moves are likely to be those that that: (i) uncover the sources, types and reasons for data non-use in a given domain; and (ii) recognise the multiple aspects to this complex issue across other domains in seeking solutions to move steadily towards socially responsible reuse of data becoming the norm. Pat's life is at stake here, and it has even been argued that harm due to data non-use is a greater risk than data misuse (St. Clair 2008). Unlike Schrodinger's pet, it is most certainly alive and manifests itself globally as a large, agile, polymorphic, lethal, black cat that must be captured and tamed.

5.15 Conclusion

Having considered some of the incongruities, dilemmas, risks and benefits in data donation, we argue that on balance it is not ethical for the vast, increasing swathes of data donated in good faith by individuals not to be used for public good. Determining what constitutes public good is another issue in itself and one that has not been explored here. It appears that, in common with other aspects of life, individuals might simultaneously hold conflicting beliefs with regards to data donation. The challenge lies in finding a bioethical balance between individual autonomy, personal exploitation and social responsibility, when our knowledge is incomplete and powerful actors have their own agendas. But to use one more analogy, let's not throw out the baby with the bathwater, but endeavour to pursue the best information we can obtain.

The demand for personal data is massive and multi-faceted, and it is in our interests to be guarded in our influences and to invest our trust with caution. Our ultimate question was whether we, as individuals and society, can make truly informed choices about data donation with the panoply of issues that may influence our decisions. This might not be a question that can be answered with a straightforward yes or no, for all the reasons we have discussed in this chapter, and more besides. It might well be impossible for any individual to comprehend the breadth of data use and its implications, but if we provide the best available information and engage properly with the information presented to us, we stand a more reasonable chance. To do that, there is an obvious need for carefully placed trust, demonstrable trustworthiness, and for Pat to hone his juggling skills.

References[8]

Allen, J., C.D.J. Holman, E.M. Meslin, and F. Stanley. 2013. Privacy protectionism and health information: Any redress for harms to health? *Journal of Law and Medicine* 21 (2): 473–485. https://www.researchgate.net/profile/Judy_Allen3/publication/260561318_Privacy_protectionism_and_health_information_Is_there_any_redress_for_harms_to_health/links/55489a9e0cf2e2031b388b1a.pdf.

Article 29 Data Protection Working Party. 2013. Opinion 02/2013 on apps on smart devices. https://autoriteitpersoonsgegevens.nl/sites/default/files/downloads/int/wp202_en_opinion_on_mobile_apps.pdf.

Beauchamp, T., and J. Childress. 2013. *Principles of biomedical ethics*. 7th ed. New York: Oxford University Press.

Cameron, D., S. Pope, and M. Clemence. 2014. Dialogue on data: Exploring the public's views on using administrative data for research purposes. http://www.esrc.ac.uk/files/public-engagement/public-dialogues/dialogue-on-data-exploring-the-public-s-views-on-using-linked-administrative-data-for-research-purposes/.

Chin, J.J.L., and A.V. Campbell. 2013. What – if anything is special about "Genetic Privacy"? In *Genetic privacy: An evaluation of the ethical and legal landscape*, ed. T.S.-H. Kaan and C.W.-L. Ho. London: Imperial College Press.

City a.m. 2017. Scottish Development International. http://www.cityam.com/261165/can-you-get-your-teeth-into-uks-322-billion-data-sector-22/3/17.

Cohen, D. 2014. Dabigatran: How the drug company withheld important analyses. *BMJ* 349: g4670. https://www.bmj.com/content/349/bmj.g4670.

Cussins, J. 2018. Direct-to-consumer genetic tests should come with a health warning. In *Beyond bioethics: Toward a new biopolitics*, ed. O.K. Obasogie and M. Darnovsky. Oakland: California University Press.

Denholm, E. 2016.Why we should worry about WhatsApp accessing our personal information. *The Guardian* (10th November 2016). https://www.theguardian.com/commentisfree/2016/nov/10/whatsapp-access-personal-information-privacy-facebook-consumers-information-commission.

Engineering & Technology. 2017. Clothing embedded with smart fabric used as digital key to open doors. https://eandt.theiet.org/content/articles/2017/11/clothing-embedded-with-smart-fabric-used-as-digital-key-to-open-doors/.

EU GDPR portal. 2018. https://www.eugdpr.org/eugdpr.org-1.html.

Farr Institute of Health Informatics Research. 2018. Data Saves Lives. http://www.farrinstitute.org/public-engagement-involvement/datasaveslives.

Foxx, C. 2018. Google and Facebook accused of breaking GDPR laws. *BBC News* (25th May 2018). http://www.bbc.co.uk/news/technology-44252327.

GeneCards. 2018. https://www.genecards.org/.

Global Alliance for Genomics and Health. 2017. Your DNA, Your Say. https://societyandethicsresearch.wellcomegenomecampus.org/sites/default/files/media/item/your-dna-your-say-at-the-global-alliance-for-genomics-and-health-plenary/files/20171017-orlando-florida-usa-ga4gh-plenary-video-of-slides.mp4.

Goldacre, B. 2013. *Bad Pharma: How medicine is broken and how we can fix it*. London: Fourth Estate publishers.

Greenbaum, D. 2018. Avoiding overregulation in the medical internet of things. In *Big data, health law and bioethics*, ed. I.G. Cohen, H.F. Lynch, E. Vayena, and U. Gasser. Cambridge: Cambridge University Press.

Gymrek, M., A.L. McGuire, D. Golan, et al. 2013. Identifying personal genomes by surname inference. *Science* 339: 321 https://pdfs.semanticscholar.org/c8f1/44712004bdfeb779b17d0b9c31e08ed2b0ef.pdf.

[8]All online references were checked, May 2018.

Haeusermann, T., B. Greshake, A. Blasimme, et al. 2017. Open sharing of genomic data: Who does it and why? *PLoS One* 12 (5). http://journals.plos.org/plosone/article?id=10.1371/journal.pone.0177158.

Hern, A. 2017. Royal Free breached UK data law in 1.6m patient deal with Google's DeepMind. *The Guardian* (3rd July 2017). https://www.theguardian.com/technology/2017/jul/03/google-deepmind-16m-patient-royal-free-deal-data-protection-act.

Herper, M. 2017. The Cost of Developing Drugs Is Insane. *Forbes* (16th October 2017). https://www.forbes.com/sites/matthewherper/2017/10/16/the-cost-of-developing-drugs-is-insane-a-paper-that-argued-otherwise-was-insanely-bad/#160396842d45.

Intersoft Consulting. 2017. EU GDPR – final text neatly arranged. https://gdpr-info.eu/.

Ipsos MORI. 2016. The One-Way Mirror: Public attitudes to commercial access to health data. Wellcome Trust. https://wellcome.ac.uk/sites/default/files/public-attitudes-to-commercial-access-to-health-data-wellcome-mar16.pdf

Jones, K.H., D.V. Ford, C. Jones, et al. 2014. A case study of the Secure Anonymous Information Linkage (SAIL) Gateway: A privacy-protecting remote access system for health-related research and evaluation. *Journal of Biomedical Informatics: Special Issue on Medical Data Privacy* 50: 196 https://www.sciencedirect.com/science/article/pii/S1532046414000045.

Jones, K.H., G. Laurie, L.A. Stevens, C. Dobbs, D.V. Ford, and N. Lea. 2017. The other side of the coin: Harm due to the non-use of health-related data. *Indian Journal of Medical Informatics* 97: 43–51 https://www.sciencedirect.com/science/article/pii/S1386505616302039.

Kalokairinou, L., H.C. Howard, S. Slokenberga, et al. 2017. Legislation of direct-to-consumer genetic testing in Europe: A fragmented regulatory landscape. *Journal of Community Genetics* 9 (2): 117–132. https://link.springer.com/article/10.1007/s12687-017-0344-2.

Laurie, G., K.H. Jones, L. Stevens, and C. Dobbs. 2015. A review of evidence relating to harm resulting from uses of health and biomedical data. Nuffield Council on Bioethics. http://nuffieldbioethics.org/wp-content/uploads/FINAL-Report-on-Harms-Arising-from-Use-of-Health-and-Biomedical-Data-30-JUNE-2014.pdf.

McCartney, M. 2017. When organ donation isn't a donation. *BMJ* 356: j1028. https://doi.org/10.1136/bmj.j1028.

Ohm, P. 2010. Broken promises of privacy: Responding to the surprising failure of anonymization. *UCLA Law Review* 57: 1701. https://www.uclalawreview.org/pdf/57-6-3.pdf.

Pencarrick Hertzman, C., N. Meagher, and K.M. McGrail. 2013. Privacy by Design at Population Data BC: A case study describing the technical, administrative, and physical controls for privacy-sensitive secondary use of personal information for research in the public interest. *Journal of the American Medical Informatics Association* 20 (1): 25 https://www.ncbi.nlm.nih.gov/pmc/articles/PMC3555322/.

Personal Genome Project. 2018. https://www.personalgenomes.org/gb.

Scott, D. 2018. Why Apple, Amazon and Google are making big health moves. https://www.vox.com/technology/2018/3/6/17071750/amazon-health-care-apple-google-uber.

Solon, O., and E. Graham-Harrison. 2018. The six weeks that brought Cambridge Analytica down. *The Guardian* (3rd May 2018). https://www.theguardian.com/uk-news/2018/may/03/cambridge-analytica-closing-what-happened-trump-brexit.

St. Clair, D. 2008. Non-use of patient clinical data a greater risk than misuse. *Managed Healthcare Executive*. http://managedhealthcareexecutive.modernmedicine.com/managed-healthcare-executive/news/non-use-patient-clinical-data-greater-risk-misuse?page=full.

Stevens, L.A., G. Laurie, C. Dobbs, and K.H. Jones. 2017. Dangers from within? Looking inwards at the role of maladministration as the leading cause of health data breaches in the UK. In *Data protection and privacy: (In)visibilities and infrastructures*, ed. R. Leenes et al. Cham: Springer International Publishing https://link.springer.com/chapter/10.1007/978-3-319-50796-5_8.

Technica UK. 2016. TOS agreements require giving up first born—And users gladly consent. https://arstechnica.co.uk/tech-policy/2016/07/nobody-reads-tos-agreements-even-ones-that-demand-first-born-as-payment/.

UK Anonymisation Network. 2018. http://ukanon.net/about-us/ukan-activities/.

UK Human Tissue Act. 2004. https://www.hta.gov.uk/policies/human-tissue-act-2004.

Ware, M., and M. Mabe. 2015. *The STM Report: An overview of scientific and scholarly journal publishing*, 4th ed. https://www.stm-assoc.org/2015_02_20_STM_Report_2015.pdf.

Wu, T. 2017. *The attention merchants: The epic struggle to get inside our heads*. London: Atlantic Books.

Part II
Governance and Regulation of Medical Data Donation

Chapter 6
Posthumous Medical Data Donation: The Case for a Legal Framework

Edina Harbinja

Abstract This article explores the options for establishing a legal framework for posthumous medical data donation (PMDD). This concept has not been discussed in legal scholarship to date at all. The paper is, therefore, a first legal study of PMDD, aiming to address the gap and shed light on the most significant legal issues that could affect this concept. The paper starts by looking at the protection of the deceased's health records and medical data, finding that this protection in law is more extensive than the general protection of the deceased's personal data, or the protection of post-mortem privacy as a concept. The paper then investigates key issues around ownership and succession of personal data, including medical and health-related data, and how these could affect PMDD and its legal framework.
The author then goes on to explore some parallels with organ donation to determine whether there are some lessons to be learned from this comparable regulatory framework. The paper concludes with the discussion around the need for a Code for posthumous medical data donation developed by the Digital Ethics Lab at the Oxford Internet Institute, and a more formal regime that would enable and facilitate this practice. Here, the author proposes key law reforms in the area of data protection and governance related to PMDD. These reforms would include amendments to the general data protection ideally, to ensure harmonisation and consistency across the EU, as well as between the general and sector-specific data protection laws and policies. These changes would contribute to legal and regulatory clarity and would help implement this important and valuable practice, which aims to facilitate research and advances in medical treatments and care.

Keywords Posthumous medical data donation · Data protection · Legal framework · Organ donation · Post-mortem privacy

---

E. Harbinja (✉)
Aston University, Birmingham, UK
e-mail: e.harbinja@aston.ac.uk

J. Krutzinna, L. Floridi (eds.), *The Ethics of Medical Data Donation*,
Philosophical Studies Series 137, https://doi.org/10.1007/978-3-030-04363-6_6

6.1 Introduction

Can individuals donate their data in life and post-mortem? In a playful and exciting episode, BBC Tomorrow's world has discussed this attractive idea, trying to invoke some of the current issues related to the use and misuse of our digital footprints and personal data.[1] Individuals are often not aware as to what happens to these digital footprints post-mortem, and the law and policy in this area are still very confusing and inconsistent (Harbinja 2017). But what if we shift this paradigm and enable users to employ their altruistic motivations and aspirations by helping them participate in 'citizen's science' and medical research through donating their medical data posthumously (Vayena and Tasioulas 2015)? This article aims to investigate the idea of posthumous medical data donation (hereinafter: PMDD) from a legal perspective, looking at what the law could do to facilitate this useful practice in the future.

The idea of PMDD is very similar to organ donation, *prima facie*. Organ donation has been a well-established topic of legal research and medical practice in many countries, including the UK (see e.g. Weimar et al. 2008; Cronin and Price 2008; Price 2000). The practice has its roots in philosophical, philanthropic and humane ideas and reasons, and the law around it has been developing in the last few decades in particular (Evans and Ferguson 2014; Skatova 2011). Data donation would have essentially a similar goal, i.e. to help save human (or other) lives and support medical and clinical practice and research. The aggregation of numerous sets of donated data would support advanced and personalised medical research, providing the basis for data mining, machine learning and AI, which would help generate new understanding of some of the acutest medical concerns that humanity is facing nowadays (e.g. cancer or various mental health conditions, Prainsack 2014).

It is important to distinguish PMDD from medical data sharing of the living, but also from medical data philanthropy, which is the opening, to access and use, by private companies and public organisations, of one's data sets, for charitable purposes (Taddeo 2016; Krutzinna et al. 2018). Krutzinna et al. argue that 'posthumous medical data donation is motivated by different reasons, and is less risky and more easily achievable than either data sharing or data philanthropy', therefore easier to implement and regulate. Importantly, the argument is that the failure to exploit fully the health data available in medical records, which often already exist in digitised form as electronic health record in the NHS, is a huge opportunity cost and has a negative effect on advancements in research. Apart from this practice being inefficient and costly, scholars argue that it is also unethical (Krutzinna et al. 2018).

In terms of individuals' readiness to engage with the option of posthumous data donation, a study finds that individuals are willing to donate personal data to research for public good, and their motivation is both self-benefit (e.g. enhancing their reputation, professional benefit, or to feel good about themselves) and concern

[1] BBC, Tomorrow's World, Donate Your Data Day, May 2018, http://www.bbc.co.uk/guides/zrh347h

for others. Surveyed individuals who were less likely to donate are motivated by self-interest mainly, whereas those more likely to donate had public good as a main motivating factor. The study concludes by arguing that 'Data Donation holds promise as a useful tool in the digital economy, providing value to third sector and well-being researchers as well as marketing and the private sector' (Skatova et al. 2014). In a different study, Jones et al. discuss what the non-use of health-related data would mean, identifying harms for the society as a whole. The study focused on issues with clinical care records, research data and governance frameworks, illustrating the types of data non-use that occur, and some of their consequences for citizens and the society (Jones et al. 2017). There is, therefore, an appetite and compelling ethical arguments for data donation more generally, as well as post-mortem. An aspect of data donation that is explored more deeply in this paper is posthumous data donation.

This article builds on the helpful findings and arguments introduced by social scientists and humanities scholars in the area (Skatova et al. 2014; Krutzinna et al. 2018; Shaw et al. 2016). One of the most tangible results of these endeavours is the Code for posthumous medical data donation developed by the Digital Ethics Lab at the Oxford Internet Institute and funded by Microsoft (Krutzinna et al. 2018). Thus, as research demonstrates, while there may be sound ethical reasons that posthumous data donation is quite straightforward, this is not necessarily the case legally. A legal framework that would support this practice has not been discussed in legal scholarship to date at all. This paper is, therefore, a first legal study of PMDD, aiming to address the gap and shed light on the most significant legal issues that could affect this concept. The focus of this paper is on the UK and English law, and the EU, where appropriate. Importantly, the study will look at the general data protection regime, *lex specialis* provision (legal regimes regulating health-related data), and data governance, thus making some useful parallels and suggestions for a reform of general and sector-specific data protection laws and policies. These changes would contribute to legal and regulatory clarity and coherence and would support the implementation and enforcement of this important and valuable practice. The legal framework would, therefore, go beyond an ethical framework that is considerably more difficult to enforce in practice.

The paper starts with a brief exploration of the current legal protection of health data and medical records in the UK more generally, and the protection of deceased's medical data and patients records, more specifically. The purpose of this overview is to ascertain if these laws and policies could apply to PMDD, or whether at least some of their principles could be borrowed for a novel PMDD legal framework. The following section looks at key issues around ownership and succession of personal data and how these could affect PMDD and its legal framework. The author then goes on to explore some overarching parallels with organ donation to determine whether there are some lessons to be learned from this comparable regulatory framework. Finally, the paper concludes with the discussion around the need for a Code for posthumous medical data donation and a more formal regime that would enable and facilitate this practice. Here, the paper proposes key law reforms in the area of data protection and governance related to PMDD.

6.2 Legal Protection of Health-Related Data of the Living and the Dead in the UK

Before analysing the law and policy around the data of the deceased, it is useful to briefly set out key data protection provisions applicable to medical and health-related data more generally, so to determine whether we could apply these to PMDD. Alternatively, the paper also investigates if we could translate provisions set out in this legislation into principles that would enable the practice of PMDD.

Health-related data in the EU and the UK have been treated as sensitive data in the Data Protection Directive 1995, and are included in the renamed category of 'special categories of personal data' in the General Data Protection Regulation 2016 (GDPR) and the Data Protection Act 2018 (DPA 2018). These data include, *inter alia*, genetic data, biometric data, and data concerning health. Processing of the special categories of data is in principle prohibited by the GDPR, and only allowed on the basis of ten general grounds, including relevant grounds for health data, such as crucially vital interests of data subject and explicit consent by the data subject (GDPR art. 9 2. (a) and (c). Further grounds are where the processing of special categories of data is necessary for the purposes of, broadly, health and social care, and for reasons of public interest in the area of public health (GDPR art. 9 2. (h) and (i). Finally, for research purposes, paragraph 2 (j) applies, and the processing of this type of personal data needs to be in accordance with Article 89(1) based on Union or Member State law. GDPR, therefore, recognises the benefits of facilitating medical research and the need for enabling the access to medical registries and data sets. This ground is relevant to medical data donation by living individuals, whereby member states are to provide for exemptions that would detail conditions and safeguards related to the processing of this data (recital 157, article 89). These specific safeguards include data minimisation, pseudonymization, and derogations from certain data subject rights, such as the right to access, to object, to rectification, to the restriction of processing. Moreover, GDPR also recognises the need for further measures in the interest of data subject and the need to apply the rules of GDPR in the light of these measures (Recital 159, GDPR). This would mean, for instance, following specific data regulatory and ethical frameworks that already exist in medical research, and could potentially include the ethical framework for PMDD. In the UK, the above provisions of GDPR have been implemented in schedule 2 part 6 of the Data Protection Act 2018 (DPA 2018).

GDPR, however, does not apply to anonymised data (see e.g. section 251 of the NHS Act 2006), so research conducted using these would not need to meet the GDPR requirements, provided that it is not possible to relate back the data to individuals, which is nowadays increasingly difficult and therefore this option should be used with caution. For anonymised data, research ethics would normally still require consent and other safeguards for data subject that are participating in a study. The further legal basis for processing of medical data in England without consent, and overriding the common law duty of confidentiality in the interests of improving patient care, or in the public interest, is set out in section 251 of the NHS Act 2006 and The Health Service (Control of Patient Information) Regulations 2002. Applications are administered by the Confidentiality Advisory Group of the Health Research Authority, but anecdotally, researchers note that the success rate is low and applicants are strongly encouraged to pursue the consent route or to use anonymous data where possible (Jones et al. 2017).

GDPR is not a helpful place to identify rules and provisions that would govern the use of the data of the deceased, including the data within PMDD. Recital 27 provides that 'This Regulation does not apply to the personal data of deceased persons. Member States may provide for rules regarding the processing of personal data of deceased persons.' Some member states have used this option and enable for the protection of the data of the deceased more generally (not limited to medical data), such as France or Hungary (see Castex et al. 2018). The UK, however, has chosen not to legislate in the area so the DPA 2018 retains the old definition of personal data, emphasising that the concept relates only to 'living individuals' (s. 3(2) DPA 2018). The fact that the GDPR and DPA do not apply directly to the data of the deceased, including posthumous medical data, makes it even more important to identify the key legal issues at play in PMDD. We, therefore, need to look beyond the general data protection framework in order to identify laws and policies that might be helpful in the context of PMDD. The next section will explore laws and policies related to the data of the deceased in the health sector, which could form a basis for the PMDD legal framework.

6.2.1 The Protection of the Data of the Deceased in the Health Sector

Sector-specific protection of deceased's medical data is somewhat more extensive than the protection awarded to the data of the deceased in the general data protection regime. For instance, The Access to Health Records Act 1990 provides for the protection of the access to health records of the deceased, and this access is permitted for 'the patient's personal representative and any person who may have a claim arising out of the patient's death' section 3 (1) f). These would be next of kin or the deceased family who might need to access these to ascertain their claims or causes of death for instance. In England, GP health records are passed on to Primary Care Support England for storage after the patient's death and these are generally retained for 10 years after death, with the exception of the storage by the Primary Care Support for England where this period extends for up to 100 years. For hospital records, the Department of Health advises that they are kept for 8 years. These are managed by the record manager at the hospital (Department of Health 2010). NHS records are also governed by the Public Records Act 1958 which provides that GP records become public when forwarded to local authorities after the death of the patient. Most of these are closed for 30 years post-mortem and those related to physical and mental health are closed for 100 years. Permission can be sought from the Public Records Office to use data from deceased persons in research if confidentiality can be guaranteed (Medical Research Council 2003). Some of the records kept longer are then opened fully to the public after this point in time.

Interestingly, the NHS data opt-out regime that allows patients to opt out from the use of their data in research, for instance, has been extended to include the data of the deceased and honouring their wish expressed premortem by the way of opting out (NHS, National Data Opt-out Operational Policy Guidance Document 2018). This policy explicitly includes deceased but does not apply if an individual has opted into a certain scheme of research by an express consent, for instance. This is a policy choice and the projection here goes beyond what is legally required by the data protection regime, as indicated earlier in this paper. Also, it provides a useful avenue for the regulation of PMDD, as opting into a PMDD scheme would exclude that data from the NHS opt-out regime. This policy, therefore, does not need to be amended in order to accommodate PMDD.

In addition to data protection, an area of law that would potentially offer a more extensive protection to deceased's patient records is the common law duty of confidence. Case law implies that the duty of confidence which doctors owe to their patients might survive the death of the patient. For instance, in *Lewis v Secretary of State for Health & Anor*[2], Mr Justice Foskett argued that a limited number of authorities in the area, including the ECHR case law and academic views, point towards this proposition. Decisions by the Information tribunal support this stance as well (see *Webber v IC and Nottinghamshire Healthcare NHS Trust*[3] and *M v IC and Medicines and Health Products Regulatory Authority*[4]). The issue is still unclear and unsettled in law, and the case law needs to be much more specific and coherent. Nevertheless, it would not be wrong to at least make a claim that this law applies to records post-mortem, even if this is an arguable point at this stage of the development of the relevant case law. As Lewis shows, the courts would also be likely to find the stance of the professional regulators and the NHS highly influential here. (see also Munns and Basu 2015). The Caldicott Review 2013 identifies this discrepancy in the law as well, calling for a legal harmonisation and for the Law Commission to ensure that there are 'no legal impediments to giving custodianship of their health and social care data within their last will and testament.' (Caldicott 2013). We will turn to this suggestion in Sect. 6.5, as it is very useful when considering a regulatory framework for PMDD. Once more going beyond the law in this area, the Department of Health, General Medical Council and other clinical professional bodies have long accepted that the duty of confidentiality continues beyond death and this is reflected in the guidance and policies they produce (Department of Health 2010).

In summary, this section identifies the most significant provisions of law and policy that could be applied to PMDD, acknowledging incoherence and the need for clarity in statutes, case law, and policies. Contrary to most types of personal data of the deceased (Harbinja 2017), confidentiality (as an aspect of a broader notion of

---

[2] [2008] EWHC 2196 (QB).

[3] GIA/4090/2012.

[4] GIA/3017/2010.

post-mortem privacy, Edwards and Harbinja 2013) of their health data and records is preserved through policy and the NHS data governance in the UK and many other jurisdictions (Shaw et al.2016). PMDD would mean that this confidentiality could be affected by the wishes of individuals expressed premortem. However, in order to make this option clear and coherent in the law, the legislation set out above would ideally need to be amended (in particular, The Access to Health Records Act 1990 and the Public Records Act 1958 would need to at least mention PMDD, so to enable the access for research purposes). Before looking at these regulatory options in more detail in Sect. 6.5, we will briefly identify some general principles around ownership and control of personal data, including medical data of the deceased. These principles and values will support and underpin the legal framework introduced later in the paper.

6.3 Some Issues Around Ownership, Privacy, Control and Succession of Data

Issues around ownership and control of data, in the context of the data of the deceased, are significant as they may influence the direction a legal regime might take, swaying it towards propertisation or away from it. It is also important to clarify the legal perspectives and discourse around property and ownership of data, as it might differ significantly from a similar discourse in social science and humanities. For example, while social scientists might use ownership and property more generally and, perhaps, imprecisely, to refer to control, it is very important not to use these in a similar manner in legal discussions and practice, for the reasons set out in this section.

Looking at a comparable legal regime, organs or body parts are not generally considered a full-blown property in law and their commercial exploitation is mostly prohibited, as discussed in the following section. Similarly, and although there have been many calls for propertisation of personal data (as there have been for different proprietary treatments of body parts), and ideas for using the doctrine of quasi-property, a predominant view in the European scholarship is that property is not an adequate legal regime to protect personal data and privacy. This regime is human rights-based and embeds values such as dignity, autonomy, control and respect for personhood. In the European legal doctrine and jurisprudence as well, it has been long established that the data protection regime is based on human rights (the ECHR and the European Charter of fundamental rights) and propertisation and commodification of personal data is not an option in any of the EU member states, including the post-Brexit UK (Harbinja 2013, 2017; Pearce 2018). Consequently, there can be no succession or bequeathing of one's data, as *stricto sensu*, only property can be passed onto one's next of kin and heirs (Harbinja 2017). An option of deciding as to what happens to one's patient records is not viable under the succession and probate regime at the moment either. Researchers argue that this is unreasonable and that there should be options for individuals to decide what happens to their data on death. (Harbinja 2017; Castex et al. 2018). This is now possible for some digital assets such as emails or social network content in France or Catalonia, however, this does not include one's medical records and data, and therefore, it is not particularly helpful as a framework for PMDD.

Due to the extremely sensitive nature of data included in patient records, it is important to consider the concept of post-mortem privacy and the protection of individuals' personal data and personality on death. In a very broad sense, post-mortem privacy includes the protection of one's body parts and organs, and the narrow interpretation includes the protection of personal data only, and thus covers patient records as well. Research shows that this phenomenon is only partially protected (Edwards and Harbinja 2013; Harbinja 2017; Buitelaar 2017) and there is not a comprehensive regime that would include data protection reform, as well as the necessary regulation of digital assets associated with the deceased's online footprints and digital persona. The UK has not followed the lead of France or the US to legislate on this matter and the DPA 2018 excludes the data of the deceased completely, as noted above. If post-mortem privacy was recognised in law, as argued by researchers, then the deceased would be able to decide as to what happens to their medical data post-mortem as well, and this would facilitate the practice of PMDD. Of course, as noted above, there may be concerns about conflicting familial interests, and any regime in relation to posthumous data donation would need to take account of this. Some suggestions proposed by Krutzinna et al. (2018) in their Code address these concerns.

Looking at post-mortem privacy from a conceptual perspective, Floridi's notion of the informational body would be significant to refer to here as well. For Floridi, a human being is constituted and exists through information related to their identity, similar to what Marx sees as the inorganic body metaphor, i.e. the idea that in producing objects, one is producing oneself at the same time. Floridian ethics emphasises the right to control one's identity, which he understands as an informational structure, constituted by everything that defines this identity, including various types of digital data. Medical and health-related data are even more closely and intimately related to one's physical body, but also concern their dignity, privacy and integrity, so the concept of informational body includes these data as well (Floridi 2013; Öhman and Floridi 2017). This theory, therefore, provides a further support for arguments against propertisation and commercial exploitation of personal data, including medical data of the deceased. This is in line with the principles and values set out in the Code for PMDD as well since the Code rejects commercial exploitation of patient's records.

The key arguments set out in the brief discussion above suggest that the legal treatment of data, inducing patients' records, is not based on property and ownership. The basis remains in human rights and personhood. Post-mortem privacy, dignity and autonomy should be used as an underlying rationale for the regime that regulates and enables PMDD. These principles do underpin the Code for PMDD, and they will form a part of an underlying rationale for a legal framework set out in Sect. 6.5. In spite of this proposition, some mechanisms of succession and probate law could be utilised to introduce and support this concept and help implement deceased's wishes. We will explore this further in Sect. 6.5.

6.4 A Comparable Regime: Organ Donation

Having argued that data is not amenable to ownership in a legal sense, we will now explore whether key legal principles of organ donation could be borrowed when designing the legal framework for PMDD. As noted in the introduction, donation of blood, organs and tissue, as well as other comparable forms of donation, share similar motivations with those that Skatova, Ng & Goulding identify for posthumous data donation of patient records and medical data (2014). The purposes of these types of donation are similar too, however, benefits might not be as obvious in the case of data donation and they may seem somewhat remote as discussed above. In law, both would be intrinsically tied to one's personhood and neither data nor body parts would normally constitute full-blown property in law, at least not the type of property that can be commercially exploited as other objects of property. There have been some instances where certain incidents of property have been assigned to body parts, but these were mainly for very specific purposes and cases, such as theft or to invoke proprietary remedies for their protection (*Doodeward and Spence*[5]; *R. v Kelly (Anthony Noel)*[6]; *Dobson v North Tyneside HA*[7]; *Yearworth v North Bristol NHS Trust*[8], The Human Tissue Act 2004, section 32; Skene 2002; Brazier 2002; Hawes 2010; Mason and Laurie 2001).

Organ donation and biomedical practices have been regulated by many international instruments (e.g. Convention on Human Rights and Biomedicine and the additional protocols to the Convention of the Council of Europe – Oviedo Convention 1997, Universal Declaration on the Human Genome and Human Rights 1997, Universal Declaration of Bioethical Principles of the United Nations 2005), as well as national statutes in the UK (The Human Tissue Act 2004, the Human Tissue (Scotland) Act 2006, Human Transplantation (Wales) Act 2013). All of these legal instruments emphasise the role of consent, either opt-in (as in England) or opt-out (or presumed opt-in, as in Wales and Scotland, see s.3 The Human Tissue Act 2004, Human Transplantation (Wales) Act 2013, the Human Tissue (Scotland) Act 2006). Consent for organ donation can be written or oral and may be given by the deceased before his death or by a third party, usually a close relative or friend.

Requirements for consent in international instruments are slightly divergent and include for instance: Oviedo Convention – free and informed, purpose explained, the right to withdraw; Universal Declaration on the Human Genome and Human Rights 1997 – free and informed consent; Universal Declaration of Bioethical

[5] 1908 6 C.L.R. 406.

[6] [1999] Q.B. 621.

[7] [1997] 1 W.L.R. 596.

[8] [2009] EWCA Civ 37; [2010] Q.B. 1.

Principles of the United Nations 2005 – prior, free, express and informed consent, adequate and the right to withdraw. All of these international treaties and declarations are based on fundamental principles of dignity, autonomy, privacy and confidentiality. In a similar form, these principles and consent requirements could be used for posthumous data donation as well, as suggested in the Code for PMDD drafted by Krutzinna et al.

There are some notable differences between organ and posthumous data donation, however. These need to be taken into account when designing a regulatory framework, as well as ethical codes. As Krutzinna et al. note, the first key difference between is the lack of physical intrusion on the donor's side in posthumous data donation. The second difference is the donor status and the lack of urgency as the utility of the data does not have an immediate expiry date in the same way as organs do. A further difference relates to the beneficiaries. Thus, while blood, cord blood and gamete donations can be used to benefit the donor in the future, in the case of posthumous data donation, the beneficiaries are always other individuals, often a group of future unknown beneficiaries of medical research. The additional important difference these researchers identify is in the research question, i.e. clinical research studies attempt to answer a specific question, whereas posthumous medical data would be used for more general research and promote curiosity in research. Researchers in traditional clinical studies will have to contact their participants if they wish to use the data for further or additional research and ask them to re-consent. This requirement does not apply in posthumous medical data donation. In addition, living participants can withdraw their consent at any point, so that their data is removed from research, the same option does not apply in posthumous medical data donation. Here, active consent management is impossible after death but could be an option premortem (Krutzinna et al. 2018). All these considerations should be taken into account when designing an adequate legal framework for this concept. For instance, there will not be an objection based on religious or ethical grounds to the use of this data, in the same way as there have been to organ donation and the integrity of a human body. For the donation for non-clinical purposes, consent will be broad but the individuals should be explained and given a choice to participate or not in this sort of research. Once opted into the scheme, the donors will not need to re-consent for further uses of their data, as long as this is broadly in line with what they consented for (e.g. the use for purely commercial purposes will be prohibited if the data is donated only for public or academic research).

There are also two risks associated with data donation, as identified by Krutzinna et al. The first one is the fact that medical data is rarely just about one individual but often relates to others, who may be harmed as a result (e.g. their family). The risk relates to the potential use that the donated data can be put to (e.g. data revealing hereditary diseased use as a basis for discrimination), thus creating a purpose creep. In these case, the researchers suggest that that particular dataset should be rejected, as it poses risks to other, living individuals. As rightly argued by Krutzinna et al., this does not dismiss the practice per se, but rather, it warns of risks researcher and stewards need to bear in mind when accepting and handling these medical records and data. In addition, safeguards already in place for medical data can be applied in the context too.

The second risk concerns the source of the donated medical data. The potential misuse of the data of the deceased naturally comes with a lower harm to the deceased as opposed to a living person, but this is also coupled with the ability to control the use of the data, which is lower in the case of the deceased's data. Krutzinna et al., therefore, suggest 'a framework that respects the values and preferences of the data donors, and that reassures potential donors that their expressed wishes will be respected after death.', pointing at concerns over the misuse of medical Big Data to justify unfair public policies, the implementation of medical profiling by employers or insurance companies etc. Any regulatory framework would need to address these too. To address these concerns and risks, these scholars propose a value-based code that would include principles and values. The code, they argue, is in line with the good practice of biomedical data schemes such as the NHS care. Data programme or the Personal Genome Project UK.

In terms of specific safeguards within the Code, which would, *inter alia*, mitigate against risks and differences between posthumous organ and data donation, Krutzinna et al. mention security, pseudonymization and encryption. It would be useful to also include safeguards such as accountability, regulatory scrutiny and transparency as required by GDPR for the use of medical data of the living in research (art. 5 and 89 GDPR, Article 29 Working Party 2018). It is argued here that specifying the need for these principles in the Code, as defined in GDPR (art. 5) and the national data protection regimes, would make the Code more robust, ethically as well as legally. Moreover, as indicated in Sect. 6.2, GDPR also recognises the need for further measures in the interest of data subject, and the Code could be perceived in the light of this provision, as it offers measures in the interest of the deceased as a data subject in the case of PMDD (notwithstanding the fact that, strictly speaking, the deceased are not data subjects under GDPR, but they could be if a member state decides so, see Sect. 6.2).

In summary, principles around organ donation and consent requirements (opt-in consent as currently required in England or presumed opt-in as in Wales; or), in particular, could be used as a blueprint for the data donation post-mortem. Any regulatory regime would need to account for risks that are different to those of organ donation, especially the one associated with a potential harm to a deceased's family and other living individuals. Consent, however, does not need to be the only or the preferred ground for post-mortem medical data donation, and considerations should be given to 'adaptive governance models' and the potentials to use public interest as a ground for this use of medical data (see e.g. Laurie et al. 2015). Relying on this ground would be arguably less complicated for the data of the deceased, as these are excluded from the general data protection regime. The sector-specific law and governance, as indicated above, however, do focus on confidentiality post-mortem, implying that consent is valuable and often required for different uses of the deceased's medical data, and the Code acknowledges this as well. We will discuss these options further in the following section.

6.5 International Framework – Code or Law?

It would be very difficult, if not impossible, to create an overarching mandatory framework for posthumous medical data donation at a global level. In the field of organ donation and biomedicine, there are numerous international instruments identified above, however, these have had limited success due to the number of signatories or the lack of enforcement in international law more generally. Therefore, an Ethical Code for Posthumous Medical Data Donation might be a better solution for an international level, where countries may choose to follow the lead of those who have already subscribed to its principles and implemented this idea successfully, to the benefit of research and science. However, as principal authors of the Code rightly argue 'it is important to regulate for the future, i.e. to avoid ethical guidelines becoming inapplicable due to technological, legal, cultural or social changes. This is the goal of the Code that we propose: to provide normative principles shaping PMDD, rather than a set of specific rules of conduct for the involved actors' (Krutzinna et al. 2018). This section will, therefore, set out some guiding principles for the legal framework for posthumous medical data donation in England, and the UK more specifically. It will also introduce basic ideas for a wider international regulation and policy.

At a European and the UK level, it is argued that GDPR would allow this practice and amendments are not strictly necessary at this point in time. Anonymised data are excluded, but also, the data of the deceased are not covered by GDPR either, nor is their protection prohibited. The lack of harmonisation opens the door to recognise initiatives like this one but also results in very disparate legal approaches across the EU. It is necessary, therefore, to utilise some of the existing sector-specific frameworks. In France, for instance, The Digital Republic Act 2016[9] could allow for this practice to be one of the specific directives made by a deceased, which is recognised by the statute. In the UK, again, DPA 2018 does not allow for the protection of the data of the deceased, so an amendment to delete the living from the definition of personal data would be helpful. However, even if the Act excludes the application of the data protection regime to the data of the deceased, there is no reason why a specific regime cannot be established as the DPA 2018 does not prohibit the protection of this data through other regimes, and we have seen above that this has been a long-standing practice in the UK health sector.

This author suggests that the legal framework only includes basic principles, such as the need for consent (opt-in or presumed opt-in), and clear exceptions where consent can be overridden, e.g. in the interests of family, where there is a case of hereditary diseases and data donation could harm others. More detailed principles for handling this process would be still set out in the Code, which would go over and beyond the existing laws, and would potentially be adopted by the NHS within their data governance structure, for instance, the NHS opt-out regime mentioned in Sect. 6.2. As indicated above, the call for an adaptive governance frameworks questions

[9] Loi n°2016–1321 pour une République numérique.

whether consent is, in fact, a 'silver bullet', and essentially refers to other grounds for processing of this data, such as public interest or research. (Laurie et al. 2015; Porsdam Mann et al. 2016). Looking at the general data protection regime, consent, in this case, is indeed not required. However, I would side with arguments put forward by the Krutzinna et al. to support the need for consent in medical data donation post-mortem. Consent, in this case, would mitigate against the caution that the Confidentiality Advisory Group expresses, as discussed above, and support the notion of post-mortem privacy. It would be helpful if the consent requirement is harmonised with GDPR, so to introduce similar standards for the protection of the deceased's medical records as those for the protection of the data of the living. As discussed earlier, however, GDPR does not apply to the data of the deceased, but it does not prevent member states from legislating in the area, so it is viable to mirror most of the consent requirements from GDPR into the PMDD framework. Consent would, therefore, need to be freely given, informed and unambiguous, by a statement or by a clear affirmative action, whereby an individual signifies agreement with PMDD. This is in line with article 4(11) of GDPR, except for it omits the word 'specific'. Researchers suggest that there could be broad and specific consent options, covering various or specific research projects and uses (Shaw et al. 2016), and the Code for PMDD suggests broad consent too. This also mirrors the consent requirements of the Universal Declaration of Bioethical Principles of the United Nations 2005, as indicated in the previous section. One could still object to this and argue that public interest in advancements in medical research overrides considerations around privacy and confidentiality. However, I would argue that highly sensitive and valuable data included in patient records still require an extent of involvement of the individual concerned. This is in line with the sector-specific regulation of deceased's health data as discussed above, including the NHS national data opt-out regime.

In terms of implementation of the principles set out above, posthumous medical data donation can also be introduced in the Law Commission's reform of wills for England and Wales (The Law Commission 2017). The deceased's decision to donate their medical data can be treated as a part of one's will, for example. Solicitors and legal profession would then be able to provide advice on these options as well. Data donor's card could be recognised similarly to the recognition of donors cards for organ donation (as suggested by the Caldicott review as well). Practically, it would also be useful to establish a register of donors in order to record wishes of the individuals centrally and avoid the need to seek consent from the families, where possible (Shaw et al. 2016). Apart from this, the Access to Health Records Act 1990 should be amended to allow for access by researchers when permitted by the deceased or their personal representative. Amendments to the NHS Act along these lines would be helpful as well. An idea would be to look at PMDD more holistically and introduce a separate regulation by the secretary of state, which would amend the relevant laws and set out the general principles of PMDD, including the recognition of ethical codes and the NHS policies. In the future, these wishes could be recorded in a third party data steward if these emerge as the new actor in the data regulatory landscape (e.g. data trusts, intelligent agents for interpreting and enforcing deceased's wishes, see similar ideas in Royal Society and British Academy 2017; House of Lords 2018).

In addition to the legal and policy changes, current technology can offer assistance in this area as well. An example is a cooperative model for managing personal health data in Switzerland, i.e. health bank and MIDATA[10]. Ther databox project in the UK could be used for this purpose as well.[11] These tools enable citizens to be in control of the storage, management and access of their personal data, including the decision how to share it and participate in citizens science (Krutzinna et al. 2018). This could be used as a tech option of recording one's wishes, however, this mechanism has to be approved by the governance model for posthumous data donation, and made sustainable and secure.

In summary, there is a clear need for principled recognition of posthumous medical data donation in law, at least at a very abstract level, through the introduction of the practice in the data protection and sector-specific legislation, which regulates the governance of medical data. The framework introduced here includes minimal legislative interventions, which could be implemented simply and quickly, without amending GDPR or DPA, for example. The options explored above include amendments to the Access to Health Records Act 1990, the NHS Act, as well as the recognition of PMDD in the law of wills. This framework aims to mitigate against potential disputes and make the practice enforceable, rather than just voluntary and code – based. An enabling and overarching framework would allow for flexibility in the implementation through ethics codes and the NHS policies. A more robust reform would include amendments to the general data protection ideally, to ensure harmonisation and consistency across the EU.

6.6 Conclusion

This paper explores the notion of posthumous donation of medical records from a legal perspective. The purpose of this paper is to initiate a broader discussion within legal scholarship and set out some overarching considerations and principles that can be applied by regulators and other stakeholders in this area.

The paper finds that the protection of the deceased's health records and medical data is more extensive than the general protection of the deceased's personal data, or the protection of post-mortem privacy as a concept. The paper also warns of some issues around ownership and succession, suggesting that regulators and researchers should refrain from referring to data being 'owned' or property in this or any other area of law, as this is incongruent with the European legal tradition, normatively and doctrinally. Hence the regulatory regime of posthumous medical data donation should be based on values and rights such as privacy, autonomy and dignity. These

[10] https://www.midata.coop/

[11] https://www.databoxproject.uk/

values have helpfully been introduced in the Code for posthumous medical data donation, for instance.

Legal framework introduced here follows the main premises of the Code, translating them into suggestions for law reforms. These reforms would include amendments to the general data protection ideally, to ensure harmonisation and consistency across the EU, as well as between the general and sector-specific data protection laws and policies. A more viable idea at this point in time includes amendments to the sector-specific law, perhaps through a separate regulation by the secretary of state for this area as well. A more light touch approach is to introduce an NHS policy that would govern this practice, akin to the NHS opt-out option from research available to the living and the dead as discussed in this paper. Finally, the law Commission should ideally consider including this option in the comprehensive reform of the law of wills they have introduced recently, so to enable individuals to records their decision about posthumous data donation in their wills or otherwise. These changes would contribute to legal and regulatory clarity and would help implement this important and valuable practice, which aims to facilitate research and advances in medical treatments and care.

Looking slightly further in the future, deceased's wishes to donate his medical data posthumously could be recorded using technological tools such as MIDATA and databox, or other forms of intelligent agents and data stewards based on machine learning and AI. However, in order to explore issues around the law, technology and human-computer interaction, a substantive, multidisciplinary future research around this idea is required, and it will be within the scope of this author's future research as well.

References

Article 29 Working Party. 2018. Guidelines on consent under regulation 2016/679. file:///C:/Users/eh14aaz/Downloads/20180416_Article29WPGuidelinesonConsent_publishpdf%20(3).pdf. Accessed 25 June 2018.

Brazier, Margot. 2002. Retained organs: Ethics and humanity. *Legal Studies* 22: 550–569.

Buitelaar, J.C. 2017. Post-mortem privacy and informational self-determination. *Ethics and Information Technology* 19 (2): 129–142.

Caldicott, Fiona. 2013. Information: To share or not to share? The Information Governance Review. https://assets.publishing.service.gov.uk/government/uploads/system/uploads/attachment_data/file/192572/2900774_InfoGovernance_accv2.pdf. Accessed 25 June 2018.

Castex, Lucien, Edina Harbinja, and Julien Rossi. 2018. Défendre les vivants ou les morts? Controverses sous-jacentes au droit des données post-mortem à travers une perspective comparée franco-américaine. *Réseaux,* forthcoming.

Cronin, J. Antonia, and David Price. 2008. Directed organ donation: Is the donor the owner? *Clinical Ethics* 3: 127–131.

Department of Health. 2010. Questions and answers about accessing health records. http://webarchive.nationalarchives.gov.uk/+/http://www.dh.gov.uk/en/Managingyourorganisation/Informationpolicy/Patientconfidentialityandcaldicottguardians/FAQ/DH_065886. Accessed 25 June 2018.

Edwards, Lilian, and Edina Harbinja. 2013. Protecting post-mortem privacy: Reconsidering the privacy interests of the deceased in a digital world. *Cardozo Arts & Entertainment Law Journal* 32 (1): 83–129.

Evans, R., and E. Ferguson. 2014. Defining and measuring blood donor altruism: A theoretical approach from biology, economics and psychology. *Vox Sanguinis* 106 (2): 118–126.

Floridi, Luciano. 2013. Distributed morality in an information society. *Science and Engineering Ethics* 19 (3): 727–743.

Harbinja, Edina. 2013. Does the EU data protection regime protect post- mortem privacy and what could be the potential alternatives? *SCRIPTed* 10 (1): 26.

———. 2017. Post-mortem privacy 2.0: Theory, law, and technology. *International Review of Law, Computers & Technology* 31 (1): 26–42. https://doi.org/10.1080/13600869.2017.1275116.

Hawes, Cynthia. 2010. Property interests in body parts: Yearworth v North Bristol NHS Trust. *Modern Law Review* 73: 130–140.

House of Lords. Select Committee on AI. 2018. AI in the UK: Ready, willing and able? https://publications.parliament.uk/pa/ld201719/ldselect/ldai/100/100.pdf. Accessed 25 June 2018.

Jones, Karina H., Graeme Laurie, Leslie Stevens, Christine Dobbs, David V. Ford, and Nathan Lea. 2017. The other side of the coin: Harm due to the non-use of health-related data. *International Journal of Medical Informatics* 97: 43–51.

Krutzinna, Jenny, Mariarosaria Taddeo, and Luciano Floridi. 2018. Enabling posthumous medical data donation: A appeal for the ethical utilisation of personal health data. *Science and Engineering Ethics*. https://doi.org/10.1007/s11948-018-0067-8.

Laurie, Graeme, J. Ainsworth, J. Cunningham, C. Dobbs, K.H. Jones, D. Kaira, and N. Sethi. 2015. On moving targets and magic bullets: Can the UK lead the way with responsible data linkage for health research? *International Journal of Medical Informatics* 84 (11): 933–940. https://doi.org/10.1016/j.ijmedinf.2015.08.011.

Mason, K., and G. Laurie. 2001. Consent or property: Dealing with the body and its parts in the shadow of Bristol and Alder Hey. *Modern Law Review.* 64: 710–729.

Medical Research Council. 2003. Ethics series: Personal information in medical research. https://mrc.ukri.org/documents/pdf/personal-information-in-medical-research/. Accessed 25 June 2018.

Munns, Christina, and Subhajit Basu. 2015. *Privacy and healthcare data: 'Choice of Control' to 'Choice' and 'Control'*. Farnham: Ashgate Publishing.

NHS. 2018. National data opt-out operational policy guidance document. https://digital.nhs.uk/binaries/content/assets/website-assets/services/national-data-opt-out-programme/guidance-for-health-and-care-staff/ndopnationaldataoptoutpolicy_v2.0.pdf. Accessed 25 June 2018.

Öhman, C., and L. Floridi. 2017. The political economy of death in the age of information: A critical approach to the digital afterlife industry. *Minds & Machines* 27: 639. https://doi.org/10.1007/s11023-017-9445-2.

Pearce, Henry. 2018. Personality, property and other provocations: Exploring the conceptual muddle of data protection rights under EU law. *European Data Protection Law Review* 4 (2): 190–208.

Porsdam Mann, S., J. Savulescu, and B. Sahakian. 2016. Facilitating the ethical use of health data for the benefit of society: Electronic health records, consent and the duty of easy rescue. *Philosophical Transactions A Mathematical Physics and Engineering Sciences.* 28: 374.

Prainsack, B. 2014. The powers of participatory medicine. *PLoS Biology* 12 (4): e1001837.

Price, D. 2000. *Legal and ethical aspects of organ transplantation.* Cambridge: Cambridge University Press.

Royal Society and British Academy. 2017. Data management and use – governance in the 21st century. https://royalsociety.org/~/media/policy/projects/data-governance/data-management-governance.pdf. Accessed 25 June 2018.

Shaw, D.M., J.V. Groß, and T.C. Erren. 2016. Data donation after death: A proposal to prevent the waste of medical research data. *EMBO Reports* 17 (1): 14–17. https://doi.org/10.1371/journal.pbio.1001837.

Skatova, A.A. 2011. *Underpinnings of higher level motivational orientations*. PhD Thesis, University of Nottingham.

Skatova, A., Ng, E., and Goulding, J. 2014. Data donation: Sharing personal data for public good?. Conference: Digital Economy All Hands Meeting. https://doi.org/10.13140/2.1.2567.8405.

Skene, L. 2002. Proprietary rights in human bodies, body parts and tissue: Regulatory contexts and proposals for new Laws. *Legal Studies* 22: 102–127.

Taddeo, M. 2016. Data philanthropy and the design of the infraethics for information societies. *Philosophical Transactions A Mathematical Physics and Engineering Sciences* 374. https://doi.org/10.1098/rsta.2016.0113

The Law Commission. 2017. Making a will. https://s3-eu-west-2.amazonaws.com/lawcom-prod-storage-11jsxou24uy7q/uploads/2017/07/Making-a-will-consultation.pdf. Accessed 25 June 2018.

Vayena, E., and J. Tasioulas. 2015. "We the Scientists": A human right to citizen science. *Philosophy & Technology* 28: 479–485.

Weimar, W., M.A. Bos, and J.J. Busschbach, eds. 2008. *The ethical, legal and psychological aspects of organ transplantation*. Lengerich: Pabst Publishers.

Chapter 7
Medical Data Donation, Consent and the Public Interest After Death: A Gateway to Posthumous Data Use

Annie Sorbie

Abstract Posthumous medical data donation (PMDD) could deliver a longitudinal dataset that facilitates significant advances in health research. This chapter focuses on a central challenge of PMDD, namely what good governance looks like in circumstances where consent does not provide a 'single magic bullet'. The central argument is that consent in PMDD must be properly understood as merely one aspect of a holistic governance regime, and that more emphasis ought to be placed on the role of authorisation. This brings to the fore the potential role of the public interest in navigating the various interests in play. As will be demonstrated, this proposed re-orientation of governance could deliver tangible benefits in PMDD and enhance three key elements of good governance: transparency, accountability and engagement with evidence of the views of actual publics. Part I outlines the impetus for the examination of PMDD in the context of the (non)delivery of the 'data sharing revolution'. Part II considers the pressure that temporal aspects of PMDD exert on traditional notions of consent, and the interests this brings into play. Finally, Part III suggests that authorisation should have a role to play alongside consent.

Keywords Posthumous · Medical · Data · Donation · Consent · Governance · Authorisation

---

The author thanks Professor Graeme Laurie for his invaluable support and advice on the drafting of this chapter. Thanks also to the Mason Institute's Work in Progress group, which commented on these nascent ideas, and in particular to Dr Edward Dove. All errors of course remain the author's own.

A. Sorbie (✉)
School of Law, University of Edinburgh, Edinburgh, UK

Mason Institute for Medicine, Life Sciences and the Law, Edinburgh, UK
e-mail: asorbie@ed.ac.uk

J. Krutzinna, L. Floridi (eds.), *The Ethics of Medical Data Donation*, Philosophical Studies Series 137, https://doi.org/10.1007/978-3-030-04363-6_7

7.1 Data Governance and the Promise of PMDD

Data use and governance is at a cross roads. Across all sectors, unprecedented quantities of data are being captured and repurposed. This is greatly facilitated by emerging technologies such as machine learning, which have transformed our capacity to analyse data in increasingly sophisticated ways (British Academy and Royal Society 2017; House of Lords Select Committee on Artificial Intelligence 2018). What may appear, at first blush, to be prosaic matters around data usage in fact require us to consider the significant (potential) benefits, and risks, of collecting, curating and sharing information beyond the purposes for which it was originally obtained or generated. As recently articulated by the British Academy and Royal Society, this raises pressing questions for society that go directly to how we live our lives and flourish in the twenty-first century.

These matters are brought into sharp focus in the context of health and the use of medical data. Here there is the very real possibility that proactive data management – whether in the form of data use, re-use or sharing – can deliver improvements in human health. However, this brings with it immediate and legitimate questions about boundaries to open science (The Royal Society 2012) and corollary responsibilities to protect data subjects and ensure good data governance (Laurie et al. 2014). The British Academy and Royal Society also highlight that while health data might tend to flow in silos, research uses might require these flows to be disrupted (and potentially significantly extended), for example where mobile phone data is used to predict the spread of malaria (Buckee et al. 2013). As well as new and varying research uses for health data, new stakeholders – including actors in the public, private and third sectors – raise questions about the public acceptability of data use and sharing initiatives that span the public / private divide (Aitken et al. 2016).

While the value and potential of data-driven medical research is well recognised (Knoppers et al. 2014) the jury is out on whether the data reuse revolution has, in fact, been delivered (Pisani and Abou-Zahr 2010). Indeed, various solutions have been proposed to bridge the gap between aspirational policy and pragmatic practice, from facilitating cross-border collaboration, to ensuring that the work invested in curating data sets is appropriately acknowledged. Despite this attention, a persistent stumbling block to progress is not so much the absence of available data, but rather how the potential of existing data might be harnessed and made available to facilitate advances in health research.

A proposal that speaks to this stubborn problem, and has attracted increasing attention in recent years, is the broad notion of data philanthropy. Taddeo (2016) understands this as 'the donation of data from both individuals and private companies'. The recipients of such data are not specified, but could include international organisations like the UN, actors undertaking research in the public sphere, or those working in industry (Taddeo 2017).

Much of the literature on data philanthropy has focused on the donation of data by private companies (Taddeo 2017). However, the donation of data by individuals has also been subject to high-profile scrutiny. In January 2018 the late British Labour MP, Baroness Tessa Jowell, delivered a speech to the House of Lords that was extensively covered by the media following her own diagnosis with a brain tumour. She called for '...sharing access to more and better data to develop better treatments' (Hansard 2018) and highlighted the work of the Eliminate Cancer Initiative (ECI). Baroness Jowell was subsequently reported to be the first to donate her medical data to the Universal Cancer Databank (BBC 2018). This kind of 'altruistic giving' is typical of many conceptions of data donation, where the language and metaphors of donation are frequently invoked to suggest admirable exercises of autonomy for the sake of the common good.

The ECI was positioned by Jowell as a new initiative, but there are now a range of data sharing schemes and repositories in operation. For example, disease specific registries, which collect information from patients, often without relying on individual consent, are well established in the UK and beyond (Nelson et al. 2016). There are also other projects, such as the Scottish Health Research Register (SHARE), which allows members of the public to voluntarily sign up to allow their coded NHS data to be checked to identify whether they would be suitable for certain health research projects, on the basis they will then be invited to participate if a match is found.[1]These projects operate in different ways, but both speak to the desire to maximise the potential of existing of health data, and to harness this to deliver collective improvements in health and social care. This too is an aim of a research project developed by Krutzinna, Taddeo and Floridi of the Digital Ethics Lab at the Oxford Internet Institute, University of Oxford, and funded by Microsoft, to investigate posthumous medical data donation (referred to hereafter as PMDD). An output of this project is to develop an ethical code for PMDD in order to set out the guiding ethical principles for such donations.

By way of context, it is only recently that there has been any sustained consideration of the use of data for research *after death* (Shaw et al. 2016). Although PMDD on a case-by-case basis might, in theory, be possible if an individual were so inclined to anticipate this before their death, there is currently no cogent framework within which such a donation may be offered up, or indeed received, and then the relevant data disseminated for research or other purposes.

To the extent that PMDD on a wider, systemic scale has previously been tentatively explored in scholarly works, this has tended to use organ donation as a comparator. Thus, an example of a potential model is Taylor's suggestion in *The Lancet* (2000) that card-carrying data donors could volunteer their data for use by brain researchers in the event that the data donor were to succumb to a brain condition. This expression of willingness to provide data would be effective in the event that a brain disorder set in, with the advantage that researchers could access information both before and after the onset of the brain illness or damage. More recently, Shaw et al. (2016) have revisited the question of how data is used after death in more detail, arguing for PMDD as a way to prevent the waste of data which might otherwise be used for valuable research. The authors identify a number of drivers of such

[1] https://www.nhsgresearchanddevelopment.scot.nhs.uk/share/ Accessed 17 August 2018.

a scheme, including: low levels of awareness of how data is used (or not) after death; the thicket of regulations that can make data from the deceased difficult to access; and the significant benefits that such use might yield, as demonstrated through the example of the German National Cohort study.

One of the assumptions of a scheme of PMDD, such as that proposed by Shaw et al. and by Krutzinna et al, is that this would be a widespread undertaking whereby individuals could, for example, opt in as a matter of course at some point in their life. Here the analogy with organ donation holds: the individual might be asked to agree to PMDD at the point where she applies for a driving licence, or perhaps signs up at a GP practice. However, for both practical and principled reasons, the organ donation analogy has significant limitations. These range from the practical matter in PMDD of locating medical records and related (but perhaps dis-located) data that may be held in different formats across multiple sites,[2] to the potential impact on living family members where shared genetic information is donated (Shaw et al. 2016 and Krutzinna et al. 2018). As will be explored later in this chapter, another divergence is that data is not exhausted by re-use in the same way as a donated organ, nor depleted by repeated use, like a biological specimen. Indeed, the longitudinal value of data potentially increases significantly over time and with increased sharing and re-use. Any effective governance mechanisms must reflect these particular features of data, its protection, and also its value maximisation.

Returning to Krutzinna et al's model of PMDD, many of the key features of this scheme are detailed elsewhere in this volume, some of which are beyond the scope of this chapter. However, the following bear repetition as they are particularly pertinent to the discussion that will follow:

- The scheme is intended to be user friendly and widespread, to encourage and enable those individuals who wish to participate to easily donate their data posthumously;
- This model of PMDD is designed to facilitate sharing of a comprehensive medical dataset, as included in participants' personal medical records (PMRs);
- Such a scheme should be voluntary and participatory – OII explicitly reject the argument that informed consent is not required for PMDD, though acknowledge the merit in further consideration of how informed consent operates where data is repurposed in ways that *cannot* be anticipated at the point of data collection. (Krutzinna et al. 2018)

This chapter responds to this call for scrutiny of what good governance looks like in circumstances where consent does not, as I will argue, provide a 'single magic bullet' (Laurie et al. 2015). The central argument advanced – that consent in PMDD should be understood as merely one aspect of a holistic governance regime – is wholly consistent with the OII's position that PMDD should enable willing

[2] This point was made by Kerina Jones of Swansea University at the OII workshop at the University of Oxford on 20th April 2018.

participants to consent to volunteer their data. However, the proposed re-orientation of governance in PMDD will further enhance the transparency and accountability of any such scheme, and support the delivery of a longitudinal dataset that has the potential to facilitate significant advances in heath research.

In the sections that follow I will first, in Part II, consider the pressures that PMDD exerts on traditional models of consent. These are analysed with reference to both the temporal regulation of PMDD, and the interests this may bring into play. This discourse serves to delineate the role of consent in PMDD, as well as its limits as a complete governance solution.

Having proposed that consent in PMDD is more properly understood as merely one aspect of a holistic governance regime, Part III suggests that authorisation has a role to play. This is where certain uses of data may be permitted by an access committee, in the absence of consent, and is illustrated by the work of the Confidentiality Advisory Group and the Public Benefit and Privacy Panel, as described further below (Laurie et al. 2015). Consideration of the operationalisation of this re-orientation, in the context of PMDD, brings to the fore the potential role of the public interest in navigating the various interests engaged.

7.2 Timing, Interests and the Limits of Consent

It is trite that issues of consent and autonomy are a central concern of health research regulation (Laurie and Postan 2013) and therefore bear scrutiny in the context of PMDD. Shaw et al. (2016) suggest that participants in PMDD would, prior to their death, be asked to provide consent for the use of their data either for individual projects, or by way of 'broad consent'. As already indicated, it is a key feature of the governance scheme proposed by OII that PMDD should operate on the basis of 'informed consent' (Krutzinna et al. 2018). In order to analyse these proposals a crucial distinction must be made between how data is donated *into* such as scheme (during a donor's life), and then collected and disseminated *out* of the scheme (once the donor is deceased). This distinction emphasises the temporal aspects of regulating PMDD, and exacerbates a frequent criticism of consent as an 'up-front, one-off event' that is unable to account for 'all interests that are in play' (Laurie et al. 2015). In the section that follows these criticisms are each examined before turning to specific models of consent.

7.2.1 A Matter of Timing

The criticism of consent as an 'up-front one-off event' has particular resonance in the context of PMDD. Here, the consent of live data donors' to the posthumous collection and use of their data is held in stasis at the point they die. This is so because there is, self-evidently, no scope to go back to the deceased donor to provide *any* information about how their data will be used, or by whom. This static consent can be contrasted with the use and value of the data provided by the donor, which proliferates over time and might be used for a multitude of research projects by a range of stakeholders in the public and commercial sectors. Given that consent to donation may come at any time prior to death, there is a considerable temporal disjuncture between the giving of consent and the use of the data; this even includes the act of collecting the data (to say nothing of its subsequent use in research) because these events will likely take place many years later. Further, and as recognised by Krutzinna et al, it is probable that, both due to the passage of time and the breadth of the information contained within a donor's PMR, the data collected will subsequently be used in ways that simply cannot be anticipated at the point of consent. This practical reality underscores the impact of the temporal aspect of PMDD governance, where the necessarily static interaction with the (dead) donor, through the medium of consent, contrasts starkly with the continuing use of the data itself. Indeed, the subject – namely the donor – is *never* temporally co-located with the object of use – the donor's data – given that this is only collected and used for research once the subject is no more.

This analysis has obvious implications for how data is donated *into* a scheme of PMDD (during a donor's life) in terms of the practical limitations of the information that can be provided to the donor at the point of consent. However, this also impacts on the operation of the scheme after the donor is deceased, and particularly on how data is disseminated *out* for use in health research. More specifically, any scheme of governance directed to the responsible dissemination of data must be able to respond to changing expectations – including those of research communities and wider publics – about how data can and should be used. The failure of the care.data initiative[3] in England provides the paradigmatic example of the perils of assuming public acceptance of new and disruptive data usages which challenge the norms of expected data flows (Carter et al. 2015; Wellcome Trust 2016). Conversely, adopting a conservative position at the point of data dissemination may be equally ethically problematic, in circumstances where participants have donated data on the understanding that this will be utilised for research.[4] The disjuncture in timing between obtaining consent and the realisation of value in data far beyond what could be anticipated at the time of consent should lead us to question seriously what informed consent could look like in these circumstances.

---

[3]This was an initiative in England that was designed to extract information from primary health records for use in secondary purposes, including research.

[4]See OII's first justification for a scheme of PMDD: that 'it is unethical to frustrate the 'will-to-do-it' without proper justification (Krutzinna et al. 2018).

7.2.2 *Interests in PMDD*

Such temporal considerations are compounded by the equally thorny criticism of consent as a governance mechanism that does not account for all of the interests in play in health research. This too calls for a 'robust assessment of what is at stake' (Laurie et al. 2015) in PMDD.

First to mind are the interests of data donors who consent (during their lifetime) to PMDD. Although these interests may be presented in different ways, few would dispute that a donor should be able to exercise their rights to self-determination or autonomy in life (Laurie and Postan 2013). On their death donors may leave behind living relatives who could also have an interest in the data that has been donated (Shaw et al. 2016). As noted by Krutzinna et al. (2018), a distinguishing feature of data is that it rarely relates to a single individual, which raises the possibility of harm to others.

At first blush the 'thicket' of regulation that applies to data relating to living individuals might appear less dense post-mortem. As was the case for its predecessor legislation, neither the General Data Protection Regulation[5] nor the Data Protection Act 2018[6] apply to information about a deceased person. However, the absence of an omnibus legislative framework does not signify a 'free for all' in terms of how the data of the deceased may be used, nor does it preclude donors' interests surviving their death. For example, Sperling (2008) argues that due respect should be given to individuals' preferences in life about how their data should be used after their death.

A growing body of scholarly work also addresses broader matters of posthumous privacy and informational self-determination (see, in particular, Buitelaar 2017; Edwards and Harbinja 2013). Buitelaar argues that the assumption that privacy rights are extinguished upon death cannot be maintained in our networked society. These matters are often considered in the context of digital assets, but many of the features of this medium, as identified by Edwards and Harbinja – such as its personal and intimate character and shareable nature – might equally be applied to electronic PMRs.

In the medical context, the persistence of obligations post mortem is reflected in guidance issued by the General Medical Council, which has long acknowledged that a doctor has a continuing duty of confidence to a patient after their death (see GMC 2018). With some equivocation, it was also found that such an obligation exists in law in the case of *Lewis v Secretary of State for Health*[7] (Choong et al. 2014). This case concerned whether documents (including medical records) relating to deceased patients could be disclosed by a GP to an inquiry into human tissue

[5] Regulation (EU) 2016/679 of the European Parliament and of the Council of 27 April 2016 on the protection of natural persons with regard to the processing of personal data and on the free movement of such data, and repealing Directive 95/46/EC (General Data Protection Regulation).

[6] c.12.

[7] [2008] EWHC 2196 (QB).

analysis in UK nuclear facilities. In *Lewis*, disclosure of the records in question turned upon whether to do so was in the public interest.[8] Here it was recognised that the public interest (which was distinguished from 'what the public found interesting')[9] was multifaceted and could encompass both individual and collective interests including those in: disclosure; maintaining the patient's confidentiality; and maintaining confidence in the institutions under investigation. [10]

This analysis again draws attention to the temporal and varying nature of the interests that may arise in PMDD, both during a donor's life when their consent is obtained, and after their death when their data is collected and used. However, here the resolution of these interests is crystallised at the point that decisions are made about how data collected by PMDD should be *disseminated out* for use in health research. Herein lies the governance dilemma at the heart of PMDD:if individual consent at the point of donation is constructed *too widely*, then this may not only stray unacceptably far beyond the intensions of the donor, it may also fail to take into account other interests that are in play, such as those of family members. However, should that original consent be construed *too narrowly*, this also risks frustrating the donor's desire to contribute to sustainable health research, in circumstances where uses go beyond what was anticipated at the time of donation, but are not necessarily unacceptable. Such a restrictive approach may also fail to take into account the full range of interests in play, including collective public interests. This leads one to question whether over-reliance on *any* model of consent is appropriate to legitimise PMDD.

7.2.3 *Models of Consent*

Questions around what constitutes an optimal model for the consent of health research participants, and the limits of that consent, have been closely and extensively scrutinised in the academic literature. There remains disagreement on terminology as between broad and blanket consents (De Vries et al. 2016) and in particular as to whether broad consent can, or cannot, be sufficiently informed in ethically robust terms (Sheehan 2011; Kaye et al. 2014). A comprehensive review of this ongoing debate falls outside of the scope of this chapter. However, briefly reviewing some potential models of consent, in light of the analysis of PMDD above – which pays close attention the subject / object disconnect and interests at play in PMDD, and also how data received *into* and disseminated *out of* such a scheme –reveals insights that can inform its good governance.

Laurie and Postan identify the 'many different qualifying adjectives' that are used to describe consent in the context of health research (2013). However, this

[8] Ibid. Paragraph 58.

[9] Ibid. Paragraph 59.

[10] The Judge's order for disclosure was explicitly subject to proper safeguards being put in place to ensure that the information did not become 'public' beyond the inquiry. Ibid. Paragraph 58. I return to further consider the role of the public interest in PMDD at Part III below.

chapter will focus on the proposals outlined by Shaw et al, and developed by Krutzinna et al, which both suggest that some form of 'broad' consent will be most appropriate in the context of PMDD, with Krutzinna et al emphasising that this should be 'informed'.[11] In the analysis of this model I will argue that, because of the temporal disconnect inherent in PMDD, and the multiple interests in play, while consent (of any type) might be a basis for signing people up to participate in PMDD, it is not well placed to be the enduring governance tool over time and certainly not after the donor's death. To the extent that such issues are a reoccurring theme in health research regulation more broadly, this is particularly so in PMDD in circumstances where the subject – the donor –is no more, while the object – the data – not only endures but proliferates over time.

Although not proposed in either of the PMDD models referred to above, I turn first (and briefly) to 'open' consent, where a donor passes over data posthumously on the basis that the recipient can 'do whatever they want with it'. This bears brief scrutiny as it could be said that this is workable *precisely because* the donor is deceased; indeed, in the case of organ donation, the donor is not consulted on exactly how that organ is used and who should be the recipient. While this analogy could appear persuasive, there are, I would argue, good reasons why this does not hold good (Shaw et al. 2016). Despite the data usage occurring post mortem, many of the ethical concerns raised in relation to open-ended consent – such as whether this could ever be meaningful or take account of the multiple interests in PMDD as outlined above –persist and are exacerbated by the multitude of ways in which the data might subsequently be used (Lunshof et al. 2008). Further, robust open consent, as operated in the context of the Personal Genome Project,[12] is a rigorous and onerous process that requires 'a high degree of 'information altruism' … thereby introducing a strong moral motive' (Lunshof et al. 2008). This might set the bar too high for many and impact negatively on rates of participation. This would be fatal to a scheme of PMDD that relies on willing data donors and aspires to a streamlined donation procedure.

This brief critique of open consent underlines why a scheme of broad consent is the scheme of choice in both PMDD proposals. For the purposes of this chapter I park the question of whether broad consent can be informed consent (see, for example, Caulfield 2007; Sheehan 2011; Kaye et al. 2014). Further, 'broad consent' itself is not an entirely settled term, and so, for expediency, I will use, as my starting point, Sheehan's (2011) understanding of this as '…encapsulat[ing] consent to a range of different conditions'. He sees this primarily as agreement to an arrangement whereby a governing body will make decisions about how data might be used,

[11] For the purposes of this chapter, I have discounted the possibility of specific consent and dynamic consent, which are clearly not possible in circumstances where a dead donor cannot be re-consented. See Kaye et al. 2014, for the benefits of dynamic consent in biobanking, as compared to broad consent. For the sake of space, and because it has not been proposed as a solution for PMDD, I have also omitted any consideration of consent by proxy in PMDD, which would occur after the donor's death.This model raises numerous ethical issues.See, for example, Wrigley (2007).

[12] See: https://www.personalgenomes.org.uk/sign-up

but notes that this can also include other matters such as 'an account of a general program of research, an account of the general goals of research or an account of the institutional values and aspirations'.

Two recent studies, both of which are broadly supportive of broad consent as a governance tool for ethical research, echo the multiple elements that broad consent encompasses. Steinsbekk et al. (2013) see broad consent as signifying acceptance of a framework to review future research, part of which includes 'strategies to update regularly the [biobank] donor' and also potentially the option of withdrawal and/or re-consenting. The authors further suggest that this interactive aspect of broad consent may be improved though the use of some of the communication methods used in dynamic consent (see also Kaye et al. 2014 for a description of this model). De Vries et al. (2016) suggest that the challenge in broad consent is to combine 'transparency about sponsored research together with governance models that assure the donor community and the public that their interests and moral concerns are being respected'. In the case of live donors to biobanks, they note that this can be achieved through access to information – for example by providing up-to-date descriptions of projects. These academic interpretations of broad consent are consistent with the recruitment, retention and access policies for UK Biobank,[13] which is recognised as operating under a scheme of broad consent. This governance model makes specific provision at the outset for 'active engagement with participants… in particular regarding the research that is being conducted on [the resource] and the research findings that emerge' (Summary), as well as incorporating provisions for the re-contact of participants in some circumstances (Section B6) and re-consent (Section B6.2).

When these recognised conditions for obtaining legitimate broad consent are considered in the context of PMDD model – where the donor's initial consent is held in stasis at the point of their death, and *no form* of ongoing interaction is possible – it could be concluded that consent is redundant in these circumstances. In particular, it fails to resolve the central governance dilemma of PMDD, as delineated above, and results in either an overreach (where this is construed *too widely*) or an under reach (where this is construed *too narrowly*), respecting neither the temporal aspects of PMDD, nor the interests in play.

Returning to the analysis above of how data is donated *into* such as scheme, as well as how it is disseminated *out* for research use, provides a more nuanced interpretation, in light of the foregoing discussion. Taking the OII scheme as our starting point, a key element of this framework is that participation should be both 'voluntary and participatory' (Krutzinna et al. 2018). In terms of the voluntariness of the donor, there is a clear role here for a scheme of broad consent as a threshold device to legitimately recruit participants *into* the scheme. For example, the donor can sign up, at the point of consent, to express their 'willingness to volunteer their data' (Krutzinna et al. 2018) within a broader governance structure. However, the analysis above also underlines the limitations of consent in the context of PMDD, when this is unable to cope with the temporal aspects of PMDD, nor the multiple interests

[13] See: http://www.ukbiobank.ac.uk/wp-content/uploads/2011/11/Access_Procedures_Nov_2011.pdf

in play, which crystallise at the point that data is *disseminated out* of such a scheme. It therefore follows that consent in PMDD is better understood as merely one aspect of a holistic governance regime, and that it is necessary to look to a range of approaches to deliver effective and enduring data governance.

So far this chapter has considered the work that different models of consent can do and concluded that, in PMDD, this will not deliver a complete solution. The circumstances of PMDD, as discussed above, preclude the discharge of some elements of broad consent, namely any form of ongoing interaction with the donor. However, some aspects of this approach, such as the review of prospective research projects by a committee to identify whether access requests should be granted to the data resource, are achievable. In the context of broad consent, this mechanism is traditionally framed as part and parcel of the consent process, effectively sitting *behind* the donor's consent. This chapter calls for a re-orientation of governance, such that consent in PMDD is more properly understood as merely one aspect of a holistic governance regime. In the section that follows I consider another potential aspect of such a regime in PMDD, namely the role of authorisation.I propose that this governance mechanism should be seen as sitting *alongside* consent. In considering how this might operate in the context of PMDD, this brings to the fore the potential role of the public interest in navigating the various interests in play.

7.3 Authorisation and the Role of the Public Interest

Authorisation is now an established, if under-researched, part of the data sharing landscape in health research (Aitken et al. 2016). Often billed as an 'alternative to consent' (Laurie et al. 2015), some of the most well-known examples that relate to data reuse are the Confidentiality Advisory Group (CAG) in England and the Public Benefit and Privacy Panel (PBPP) in Scotland. To provide some context, CAG is a statutory body[14] that advises the Health Research Authority on requests to access NHS patient records without consent for research purposes.[15]CAG's legislative framework allows the common law duty of confidentiality to be lifted in specified circumstances so that identifiable information may be shared for purposes, including medical research. There are various safeguards within the legislation, one of which is that the activity in question must be in the public interest or in the interests of improving patient care. In Scotland, PBPP has a similar mandate in terms of scrutinising requests to use NHS Scotland-controlled data, and some data controlled by the Registrar General, for research or specified 'other' purposes.[16]In contrast to its English counterpart, PBPP does not operate on a legislative basis, but rather as

[14]The CAG discharges its function pursuant to Section 251 of the National Health Services Act 2006, and The Health Service (Control of Patient Information) Regulations 2002.

[15]See: https://www.hra.nhs.uk/about-us/committees-and-services/confidentiality-advisory-group/legal-frameworks/

[16]See: http://www.informationgovernance.scot.nhs.uk/pbpphsc/

part of the governance structure of NHS Scotland. The public interest – including that both in protecting individual privacy and in optimising the use of health and social care data – is at the heart of PBPP's guiding principles. As a result, any request for access to either of these data resources must first show, amongst other matters, that the proposed use is demonstrably in the public interest.

For both CAG and PBPP, authorisation as a governance mechanism is invoked on the basis that neither consent nor anonymisation are appropriate or practicable (Aitken et al. 2016). How, then, might a scheme of authorisation work *alongside* consent to meet some of the governance challenges that are specific to PMDD? There are, as outlined below, tangible benefits this could deliver to PMDD in order to enhance three key elements of good governance: transparency, accountability and engagement with evidence of the views of actual publics.

First, by viewing the authorisation mechanism as sitting *alongside* consent, this will provide donors with a more realistic and informed understanding, at the point of consent, of how their data will be managed in the future, and particularly after their death. This re-orientation of governance, in response to the context of PMDD, explicitly acknowledges the temporal disconnect identified in this chapter as between the subject – being the donor who consents to the data donation in life – and the object – being the multitude of ways that the data may be used after the donor's death. This shift therefore delivers greater transparency in relation to the work that broad consent *can* do as a threshold device, while acknowledging that, on death, the donor is effectively handing over control of their data to the PMDD scheme and its longitudinal governance mechanism.

Next, such a mechanism, which I propose should regulate the dissemination of data on the basis that access will only be granted where this is in the public interest,[17] would potentially be capable of accounting for the multiple individual and collective interests at play in PMDD (British Academy and The Royal Society 2017). In the course of the preceding discussion, various interests in PMDD have been identified, including those of: donors (both pre and post mortem); family members; funders and researchers in the academic, commercial and third sectors; as well as the collective interests of wider publics in the benefits of responsible health research. As has been acknowledged, consent is able to take into account some of these interests, particularly in relation to the individual interests of the donor, but is inadequate to deliver upon all of the interests that are in play (Laurie et al. 2015).

In proposing demonstrable public interest as the basis on which access to data will, or will not, be granted, it is fair to acknowledge this remains a 'notoriously uncertain idea' in health research regulation (Taylor 2011), which requires further intellectual scrutiny (see various commentators in Sorbie 2016). The parameters of

[17] Shaw et al. do not go into the detail of such a governance mechanism, while Krutzinna et al. propose that access decisions should be made on the basis of the common good. I favour the public interest as this reflects the practice of established governance mechanisms (e.g. CAG, PBPP and UK Biobank) and reflects 'the importance of ensuring that data uses align with public interests or preferences' (Aitken et al. 2016). This scrutiny of the role of the public interest in health research regulation is addressed more specifically in my doctoral research.

this chapter do not allow for this task to be executed in detail, save to tease out the contours of a *holistic* conception of the public interest that might lend itself to the governance challenges of PMDD. In particular, this moves away from a narrow account of the public interest that pits individual interests against collective benefits, and towards an account that is described by Rid as a 'pluralistic conception of public interest', i.e. an account that is capable of recognising that multiple interests are in play (in particular, see Rid and Taylor in Sorbie 2016). This approach is evident both in the operation of CAG and PBPP,[18] and is in line with the judicial interpretation of a multifaceted public interest in *Lewis*. The operation of a similar scheme can be seen in the case of the UK Biobank, which uses the public interest to regulate third party access to its resource (Capps 2012). However, PMDD, which only collects and disseminates data in the future once its donors are deceased, can be distinguished from most biobanks, whose aim is to create a more immediate resource, often for use during a donor's lifetime.

Third, an authorisation mechanism, which allows access to data gathered by PMDD when this is in the public interest, has the potential to connect the governance of a scheme of PMDD, with the mounting empirical evidence of public attitudes towards data sharing and linkage, thus closing the gap between aspirational policy and pragmatic practice. This chapter has already touched on the perils of disregarding the need for a 'social licence' for any such scheme, and the need to tread carefully in the case of new, and potentially disruptive, data flows. This is also illustrated in Wellcome's recent research, as commissioned from Ipsos MORI, on public attitudes to commercial access to health data for research purposes (Wellcome Trust 2016). This found that, when considering data uses, 'a strong case for public benefit is the most important factor for many people: without it, data use by any organisation is rarely acceptable'. While these findings did not relate specifically to PMDD, this is particularly relevant in the context of a scheme that relies on a voluntary and participatory model, as without wiling data donors, the scheme will fail before it begins.

Given that authorisation schemes are an established part of the data sharing landscape, Aitken et al.'s finding that there is a lack of evidence of public views on this topic is striking. The conclusions of this chapter certainly suggest that further scrutiny of authorisation as a governance mechanism is likely to have wide application, reaching beyond the current modes in which this is deployed. In the case of PMDD, any proposed governance model would be well-advised to undertake a comprehensive public engagement exercise to gauge both understandings of access decisions that are made in the public interest, and also the extent to which this might be tolerated by publics. In shaping the contours of how a consent and authorisation model might work in tandem, this exercise could explore matters such as whether authorisation should always seek to take donors' early consent into account, the extent to which

[18] For example, the Terms of Reference for the PBPP explicitly recognise that: 'To ensure the right balance is struck between safeguarding the privacy of all people in Scotland and the fiduciary duty of Scottish public bodies to make the best possible use of the health and social care data collected – it is important to note that each is in the public interest'. See: http://www.informationgovernance.scot.nhs.uk/pbpphsc/home/about-the-panel/

donors should be able to place conditions on the use of their data, and whether there could ever be circumstances, such as the passage of time, that would legitimately allow an authorisation mechanism to allow access to data in the public interest that goes beyond the scope of the original consent.

7.4 Conclusion

PMDD is a proposal that speaks directly to the persistent challenge of harnessing *existing* data in order to facilitate future research, and holds the promise of delivering significant advances in human health. This chapter has scrutinised what good governance looks like in circumstances where, as I have argued, consent does not provide a 'single magic bullet' (Laurie et al. 2015).

This central argument – that consent in PMDD must be properly understood as merely one aspect of a holistic governance regime, and that more emphasis ought to be placed on the role of authorisation – has brought to the fore the potential role of the public interest in navigating the various interests in play in the context of PMDD. This chapter has further set out how a re-orientation of governance could deliver tangible benefits to the good governance of PMDD, thus enhancing its transparency, accountability and engagement with evidence of the views of actual publics.

This chapter contributes to the growing literature on PMDD by elucidating the impact of temporal regulation on good governance in this context, where the necessarily static interaction with the (dead) donor, through the medium of consent, contrasts starkly with the continuing use of the data itself. Indeed, it has been highlighted that the subject – namely the donor – is *never* temporally co-located with the object of use – the donor's data – given that this is only collected and used for research once the subject is no more. This analysis has also highlighted the need to account for multiple individual and collective interests at play in PMDD that are likely to change over time. Taken together, this points to the need for an adaptive governance model that is reoriented to meet the specific challenges of PMDD, and thus provides a gateway to posthumous medical data use.

These contributions also have wider application in health research regulation that go beyond PMDD. In particular, this chapter proposes a framework to analyse innovative data governance regimes with reference to how data flows *into*, and is disseminated *out of*, these models. By highlighting temporal considerations in health research regulation, and the multiple individual and collective interests engaged, this underlines the need for novel and bold mechanisms that do not seek to over-play the role of consent, nor that suggest that third party permissions alone can deliver good governance solutions. Dynamic governance that captures the strengths of each of these approaches is required to bring about a crucial step-increase in health research capabilities when it comes to dealing respectfully and effectively with data after death.

References

Aitken, Mhairi, Jenna de St. Jorre, Clausia Pagliari, Ruth Jepson, and Sarah Cunningham-Burley. 2016. Public responses to the sharing and linkage of health data for research purposes: A systematic review and thematic synthesis of qualitative studies. *BMC Medical Ethics* 17 (73). https://doi.org/10.1186/s12910-016-0153-x.

BBC. 2018. *Ex-MP Tessa Jowell first to donate data to medical database*. 20 April. https://www.bbc.co.uk/news/uk-politics-43833022. Accessed 21 June 2018.

British Academy and the Royal Society. 2017. *Data management and use: Governance in the 21st century*. https://royalsociety.org/~/media/policy/projects/data-governance/data-management-governance.pdf. Accessed 21 June 2018.

Buckee, Caroline, Amy Wesolowski, Nathan Eagle, Elsa Hansen, and Robert W. Snow. 2013. Mobile phones and malaria: Modelling human and parasite travel. *Travel Medicine and Infectious Disease* 11 (1): 15–22.

Buitelaar, J.C. 2017. Post-mortem privacy and informational self-determination. *Ethics and Information Technology* 19 (2): 129–142.

Capps, Benjamin. 2012. The public interest, public goods, and third-party access to UK Biobank. *Public Health Ethics* 5 (3): 240–251.

Carter, Pam, Graeme Laurie, and Mary Dixon-Woods. 2015. The social licence for research: why care.data ran into trouble. *J Med Ethics* 41: 404-409.

Caulfield, Timothy. 2007. Biobanks and blanket consent: The proper place of the public good and public perception rationales. *King's Law Journal* 18: 209–226.

Choong, Kartina Aisha, Mifsud Bonnici, and Jeanna Pia. 2014. Posthumous medical confidentiality: The public interest conundrum. *European Journal of Comparative Law and Governance* 1: 106–119.

De Vries, Raymond Gene, Tom Tomlinson, Hyungjin Myra Kim, Chris Krenz, Diana Haggerty, Kerry A. Ryan, and Scott Y.H. Kim. 2016. Understanding the public's reservations about broad consent and study-by-study consent for donations to a biobank: Results of a national survey. *PLoS One* 11 (7). https://doi.org/10.1371/journal.pone.0159113.

Edwards, Lilian, and Edina Harbinja. 2013. Protecting post-mortem privacy: Reconsidering the privacy interests of the deceased in a digital world. *Cardozo Arts and Entertainment Law Journal* 32: 83–129.

General Medical Council. 2018. Confidentiality: good practice in handling patient information. https://www.gmc-uk.org/ethical-guidance/ethical-guidance-for-doctors/confidentiality/managing-and-protecting-personal-information. Accessed 21 June 2018.

House of Lords Select Committee on Artificial Intelligence, Report of Session 2017–19. 2018. *AI in the UK: Ready, willing and able?* https://publications.parliament.uk/pa/ld201719/ldselect/ldai/100/100.pdf. Accessed 1 Aug 2018.

Jowell, Tessa. 2018. Hansard. 778: 1169–1170. https://hansard.parliament.uk/lords/2018-01-25/debates/2665383A-7D07-42B2-8DA0-581D43365F2D/NHSCancerTreatments#1170. Accessed 21 June 2018.

Kaye, Jane, Edgar A. Whitley, David Lund, Michael Morrison, Harriet Teare, and Karen Melham. 2014. Dynamic consent: A patient interface for twenty-first century research networks. *European Journal of Human Genetics* 23: 141–146.

Knoppers, Bartha, Jennifer Harris, Isabelle Budin-Ljøsne, and Edward Dove. 2014. A human rights approach to an international code of conduct for genomic and clinical data sharing. *Human Genetics* 133 (7): 895–903.

Krutzinna, Jenny, Mariarosaria Taddeo, and Luciano Floridi. 2018. Enabling posthumous medical data donation: A appeal for the ethical utilisation of personal health data. *Science and Engineering Ethics*. https://doi.org/10.1007/s11948-018-0067-8.

Laurie, Graeme, and Emily Postan. 2013. Rhetoric or reality: What is the legal status of the consent form in health-related research? *Medical Law Review* 21: 371–414.

Laurie, Graeme, Leslie Stevens, Kerina Jones, and Christine Dobbs. 2014. *A review of evidence relating to harm from uses of health and biomedical data*. Nuffield Council on Bioethics. http://

nuffieldbioethics.org/wp-content/uploads/A-Review-of-Evidence-Relating-to-Harms-Resulting-from-Uses-of-Health-and-Biomedical-Data-FINAL.pdf. Accessed 21 June 2018.

Laurie, G., J. Ainsworth, J. Cunningham, C. Dobbs, K. Jones, D. Kaira, N.C. Lea, and N. Sethi. 2015. On moving targets and magic bullets: Can the UK lead the way with responsible data linkage for health research? *International Journal of Medical Informatics* 84 (11): 933–940. https://doi.org/10.1016/j.ijmedinf.2015.08.011.

Lunshof, Jeantine E., Ruth Chadwick, Daniel B. Vorhaus, and George M. Church. 2008. From genetic privacy to open consent. *Nature Reviews Genetics* 9: 406–411. https://doi.org/10.1038/nrg2360.

Nelson, Eugene, Mary Dixon-Woods, Paul B. Batalden, Karen Homa, Aricca D. Van Citters, Tamara S. Morgan, Elena Eftimovska, Elliott S. Fisher, John Ovretveit, Wade Harrison, Cristin Lind, and Staffan Lindblad. 2016. Patient focussed registries can improve health, care and science. *BMJ* 354: i3319.

Pisani, Elizabeth, and Carla Abou-Zahr. 2010. Sharing health data: Good intentions are not enough. *Bulletin of the World Health Organization* 88 (6): 462–466.

Shaw, David, Juliane Gross, and Thomas Erren. 2016. Data donation after death. *EMBO Reports* 17: 14–17.

Sheehan, Mark. 2011. Can broad consent be informed consent? *Public Health Ethics* 4 (3): 226–245.

Sorbie, Annie. 2016. Conference report: Liminal spaces symposium at IAB 2016: What does it mean to regulate in the public interest? *SCRIPT-ed* 13 (3): 375–381.

Sperling, Daniel. 2008. *Posthumous Interests: Legal and Ethical Perspectives*. Cambridge: Cambridge University Press.

Steinsbekk, Kristin Solum, Bjørn Kare Myskja, and Berge Solberg. 2013. Broad consent versus dynamic consent in biobank research: Is passive participation an ethical problem? *European Journal of Human Genetics* 21: 897–902.

Taddeo, Mariarosaria. 2016. Data philanthropy and the design of the infraethics for information societies. *Philosphical Transactions of the Royal Society* 374: 2083.

———. 2017. Data philanthropy and individual rights. *Minds & Machines* 27: 1–5.

Talylor, Kathleen. 2000. A data-donor scheme for brain researchers. *The Lancet* 355: 849–850.

Taylor, Mark. 2011. Health research, data protection, and the public interest in notification. *Medical Law Review* 19: 267–303.

The Royal Society. 2012. *Science as an open enterprise*. https://royalsociety.org/~/media/policy/projects/sape/2012-06-20-saoe.pdf. Accessed 21 June 2018.

Wellcome Trust. 2016. *The one-way mirror: Public attitudes to commercial access to health data*. https://wellcome.ac.uk/sites/default/files/public-attitudes-to-commercial-access-to-health-data-wellcome-mar16.pdf. Accessed 24 June 2018.

Wrigley, Anthony. 2007. Proxy consent: Moral authority misconceived. *Journal of Medical Ethics* 33: 527–531.

Part III
Implementing Ethical Medical Data Donation

Chapter 8
The Personal Data Is Political

Bastian Greshake Tzovaras and Athina Tzovara

Abstract The success of personalized medicine does not only rely on methodological advances but also on the availability of data to learn from. While the generation and sharing of large data sets is becoming increasingly easier, there is a remarkable lack of diversity within shared datasets, rendering any novel scientific findings directly applicable only to a small portion of the human population. Here, we are investigating two fields that have been majorly impacted by data sharing initiatives, neuroscience and genetics. Exploring the limitations that are a result of a lack of participant diversity, we propose that data sharing in itself is not enough to enable a global personalized medicine.

Keywords Genetics · Personalized medicine · Neuroscience · Data sharing · Diversity · Open data · Machine learning

8.1 Introduction

Personalized or stratified medicine has been one of the hot topics in health care, reaching well beyond the launch of the Precision Medicine Initiative in the United States (Collins and Varmus 2010). The promise of personalized medicine is to identify individuals at risk and find optimally tailored health care solutions based on their genetic and environmental makeup (Lu et al. 2014). Although personal medicine spans over a variety of medical and biological disciplines, two subfields are particularly promising due to their growing adoption: genetics and neuroscience. Indeed, many current examples of precision medicine come from pharmacogenomics in general, specifically from oncology, where cancer treatments are picked to

B. Greshake Tzovaras (✉)
Lawrence Berkeley National Laboratory, Berkeley, CA, USA

Open Humans Foundation, Sanford, NC, USA

A. Tzovara
Helen Wills Neuroscience Institute, University of California, Berkeley, CA, USA

J. Krutzinna, L. Floridi (eds.), *The Ethics of Medical Data Donation*,
Philosophical Studies Series 137, https://doi.org/10.1007/978-3-030-04363-6_8

match the mutations found in tumours (Kummar et al. 2015; Smith 2012; Tan and Du 2012).

While this use of genetic data in health care is projected to become more central in the next years, its success will depend on multiple factors. As for most things in healthcare, cost plays a huge role. But while the costs for performing a high precision medical examination, like a brain scan, or sequencing a human genome continue to drop (Wetterstrand 2018), their usefulness is bound by both our ability to quickly process these large amounts of data as well as the lack of medically-relevant scientific knowledge we have about individual genetic variants (Dewey et al. 2014), or complex neurobiological processes. As such it is key that science be able to generate genetic knowledge more quickly (Kohane 2015).

Two recent trends in science, big data and artificial intelligence, appear to be promising for not only accelerating our genomic and neurobiological understanding but also for diagnosing in a precision medicine framework (Moon et al. 2007; Dilsizian and Siegel 2014). The idea is that artificial intelligence can be used to mine large data sets to find the smallest associations between genetic variants / neuromarkers and disease phenotypes, and to track disease progression or predict optimal treatments. To effectively create such large data collections it thus becomes central to link and share individual data sets (Kohane 2015). But while the total number of basepairs sequenced per time as well as the total number of participants included in neuroscientific studies have exponentially increased over the last years, sharing practices for such data has not kept up a similar speed (Kovalevskaya et al. 2016), despite individual efforts to enable open sharing of genetic (Mao et al. 2016; Greshake et al. 2014) or neuroscientific (Poline et al. 2012) data.

8.2 Sharing Genomic Data

To alleviate these shortcomings individual academic consortia have been founded to pool data sets across institutions and individual researchers. National efforts include the *UK10K* ("UK10K" 2018), which aimed to sequence 10,000 participants in the United Kingdom and the similarly structured *100,000 Genomes Project* by *Genomics England* ("Genomics England" 2018). In the United States, the *Exome Aggregation Consortium* (ExAC) ("ExAC" 2018) – which has collected over 60,000 exomes - and more recently the *All of Us* initiative ("All of Us" 2018) are collecting and aggregating more patient data for research purposes. And it is not only academic research that is starting to collect large data sets for personalized medicine, commercial companies are starting to explore the field too.

Since *deCODE Genetics* and *23andMe* released the first Direct-To-Consumer genetic tests back in 2007 (Vorhaus 2010), the market for commercial genetic testing has grown significantly: Not only in terms of companies like *MyHeritage*, *FamilyTreeDNA*, *AncestryDNA* or *Veritas* that have entered the market, but also in terms of the number of people who have gotten genetic tests through these services. Today, *AncestryDNA* has over five million customers and industry veteran *23andMe* has genetic data for over two million people (McAllister 2017). These sizable commercial databases are of interest to academic and commercial researchers. *23andMe* has collaborated with academic researchers on numerous research papers ("23andMe Research" 2018) and has done commercial for-profit collaborations with pharmaceutical companies like *Pfizer* and *Genentech.*

Who profits from such large-scale research remains open. As an example, in psychology the need to look into how representative study participants are has been acknowledged. After all, around 80% of all participants in psychology studies are from WEIRD (Western, Educated, Industrialized, Rich, Democratic) countries and do thus not represent human diversity (Henrich et al. 2010). As such, only WEIRD participants can fully profit from much of psychological research. To avoid the over-representation of WEIRD individuals found in psychology, it is key that our genetic research data resources reflect human diversity across populations. Indeed, this issue of representativeness becomes even more central in the genetic framework of Genome Wide Association Studies (GWAS). These studies are commonly used to inform personalized medicine by identifying genetic risk factors, e.g. for cancer (Agyeman and Ofori-Asenso 2015). Unfortunately, most of these identified risk factors are mere correlations, not genes directly causing a disease. As these correlations depend on the ancestry context in which they were found, findings of a GWAS are not necessarily applicable outside the human population in which an association was initially found (Bush et al. 2012) and cannot be replicated in many cases (Marigorta et al. 2013).

Indeed, many data sharing efforts show such a lack of population diversity: More than 50% of the over 60,000 samples in the ExAC consortium come from a European population ("ExAC" 2018). Similarly, commercial databases like the ones of *23andMe* suffer from ancestry and race biases ("Problems with 23andMe Ancestry Composition" 2015; Euny Hong 2016). Open genomic databases – like the Personal Genome Projects and openSNP – are not fairing much better: 75% of participants in one of Harvard's Personal Genome Project studies identified as white (Mao et al. 2016) and amongst a survey of over 500 openSNP participants over 70% come from the US, UK and Canada. Additionally, over 75% of openSNP participants had at least a Bachelor's degree, hinting at a highly skewed demographic (Haeusermann et al. 2017).

8.3 Sharing Neurobiological Data

Similar to genetics, neuroscience has gone a long way when it comes to data sharing: While initial attempts to share data mainly focused on post-processed data, like coordinate-based results or statistical maps of magnetic resonance imaging (MRI) (Fox and Lancaster 2002), more recent initiatives enable sharing of entire functional or structural MRI datasets (Gorgolewski et al. 2015; Poldrack et al. 2013) and magneto- or electro- encephalography (M/EEG) data (Niso et al. 2016).

As in the case of psychology and genomics, neuroscience research is largely based on data of individuals from WEIRD societies (Falk et al. 2013), despite a plethora of studies showing that brain development is affected by socioeconomic status, early life stress, or cultural differences (Hackman et al. 2010; Marshall et al. 2018; Chan et al. 2018; Duval et al. 2017; Liddell and Jobson 2016). Indeed, within or across household socio-economic variables during childhood, such as family income, parental education (Ellwood-Lowe et al. 2018; Weissman et al. 2018) or neighbourhood poverty levels (Marshall et al. 2018), can be traced on trajectories of brain development, and result in differences in brain structure (Ellwood-Lowe et al. 2018) and cognitive functions (Hackman and Farah 2018), or gene expression (Parker et al. 2017). Differences in brain networks according to socio-economic status are also evident during adolescence (Weissman et al. 2018) and adulthood (Chan et al. 2018).

Furthermore, culture has been shown to influence neural functions (Liddell and Jobson 2016). Cultural and ethnic differences have an impact on emotion perception and expression, and brain responses to emotional or social cues (Derntl et al. 2012). Moreover, ethnic differences have been found in physiological responses to fear or novelty (Martínez et al. 2014; Kredlow et al. 2017), which are commonly used to assess anxiety or post-traumatic stress disorders (Bach et al. 2017). This situation is aggravated by the fact that ethnicity can influence skin conductance responses (Kredlow et al. 2017), which are commonly used as laboratory measurements of fear mechanisms (Tzovara et al. 2018), potentially leading to the exclusion of ethnicities despite being at higher risk e.g. for post-traumatic stress disorders (Roberts et al. 2011).

How much existing data sharing efforts for neuroscience are affected by these biases is hard to estimate at this point: Although these initiatives generally tend to support standardized data formats for data sharing (Niso et al. 2018; Gorgolewski et al. 2016), they only rarely include concrete guidelines for reporting of socio-demographic variables (Madan 2017).

8.4 Data Sharing as a Social Movement

All of this paints a bleak picture: The populations we are using to develop personalized medicine are highly WEIRD (Henrich et al. 2010). Even worse, we might often not even be aware of this, as we are not collecting the needed demographic data to identify our biases. Depending on the field, research studies can furthermore only contain small sample sizes, making it hard to evaluate how ethnicity or social factors influence neurobiological functions and gene expression. Only by sharing diverse datasets, and including rich demographic information will it be possible to make our understanding of disease progression, and neurobiological functions relevant for all individuals, irrespective of their social or ethnic background.

Back in 2005, Thomas Friedman firmly believed that *next great breakthrough in bioscience could come from a 15-year-old who downloads the human genome in Egypt* (Pink 2005). Today, we have to acknowledge that there is a good chance that this 15-year-old would not be able to profit from their own breakthrough. Because of this, we are still far away from a truly personalized medicine, making our personal data political. It is up to us, the generators of data and the people sharing data to work on changing this, ensuring that the promise of personalized medicine is equitable. Or to say it with Carol Hanisch's words: *There are no personal solutions at this time. There is only collective action for a collective solution* (Hanisch 1969).

References

"23andMe Research". 2018. https://research.23andme.com/publications/.

Agyeman, AkosuaAdom, and Richard Ofori-Asenso. 2015. Perspective: Does personalized medicine hold the future for medicine? *Journal of Pharmacy and Bioallied Sciences* 7 (3): 239. https://doi.org/10.4103/0975-7406.160040.

"All of Us". 2018. https://allofus.nih.gov.

Bach, D.R., A. Tzovara, and J. Vunder. 2017. Blocking human fear memory with the matrix metalloproteinase inhibitor doxycycline. *Molecular Psychiatry* 23: 1584–1589. https://doi.org/10.1038/mp.2017.65.

Bush, William S., Jason H. Moore, J. Li, S.K. McDonnell, and K.G. Rabe. 2012. Chapter 11: Genome-wide association studies. *PLoS Computational Biology* 8 (12): e1002822. https://doi.org/10.1371/journal.pcbi.1002822.

Chan, Micaela Y., Jinkyung Na, Phillip F. Agres, Neil K. Savalia, Denise C. Park, and Gagan S. Wig. 2018. Socioeconomic status moderates age-related differences in the Brain's functional network organization and anatomy across the adult lifespan. *Proceedings of the National Academy of Sciences of the United States of America* 115: E5144–E5153. https://doi.org/10.1073/pnas.1714021115.

Collins, Francis S., and Harold Varmus. 2010. A new initiative on precision medicine. *Perspective* 363 (1): 1–3. https://doi.org/10.1056/NEJMp1002530.

Derntl, Birgit, Ute Habel, Simon Robinson, Christian Windischberger, Ilse Kryspin-Exner, Ruben C. Gur, and Ewald Moser. 2012. Culture but not gender modulates amygdala activation during explicit emotion recognition. *BMC Neuroscience* 13 (1): 54. https://doi.org/10.1186/1471-2202-13-54.

Dewey, Frederick E., Megan E. Grove, Cuiping Pan, Benjamin A. Goldstein, Jonathan A. Bernstein, Hassan Chaib, Jason D. Merker, et al. 2014. Clinical interpretation and implications of whole-genome sequencing. *JAMA – Journal of the American Medical Association* 311 (10): 1035–1044. https://doi.org/10.1001/jama.2014.1717.

Dilsizian, Steven E., and Eliot L. Siegel. 2014. Artificial intelligence in medicine and cardiac imaging: Harnessing big data and advanced computing to provide personalized medical diagnosis and treatment. *Current Cardiology Reports* 16 (1). https://doi.org/10.1007/s11886-013-0441-8.

Duval, Elizabeth R., Sarah N. Garfinkel, James E. Swain, Gary W. Evans, Erika K. Blackburn, Mike Angstadt, Chandra S. Sripada, and Israel Liberzon. 2017. Childhood poverty is associated with altered hippocampal function and visuospatial memory in adulthood. *Developmental Cognitive Neuroscience* 23: 39–44. https://doi.org/10.1016/j.dcn.2016.11.006.

Ellwood-Lowe, Monica E., Kathryn L. Humphreys, Sarah J. Ordaz, M. Catalina Camacho, Matthew D. Sacchet, and Ian H. Gotlib. 2018. Time-varying effects of income on hippocampal volume trajectories in adolescent girls. *Developmental Cognitive Neuroscience* 30: 41–50. https://doi.org/10.1016/j.dcn.2017.12.005.

Euny Hong. 2016. *23andMe has a problem when it comes to ancestry reports for people of color*. 2016.

"ExAC". 2018. http://exac.broadinstitute.org/faq.

Falk, Emily, Hyde Luke, Colter Mitchel, Jessica Faul, and Et. Al. 2013. What is a representative brain? Neuroscience meets population science. *PNAS* 110 (44): 17615–17622.

Fox, Peter T., and Jack L. Lancaster. 2002. Mapping context and content: The BrainMap model. *Nature Reviews Neuroscience* 3 (4): 319–321. https://doi.org/10.1038/nrn789.

Genomics England. 2018. https://www.genomicsengland.co.uk/.

Gorgolewski, Krzysztof J., Gael Varoquaux, Gabriel Rivera, Yannick Schwarz, Satrajit S. Ghosh, Camille Maumet, Vanessa V. Sochat, et al. 2015. NeuroVault.org: A web-based repository for collecting and sharing unthresholded statistical maps of the human brain. *Frontiers in Neuroinformatics* 9. https://doi.org/10.3389/fninf.2015.00008.

Gorgolewski, Krzysztof J., Vince D. Tibor Auer, R. Cameron Craddock Calhoun, Samir Das, Eugene P. Duff, Guillaume Flandin, et al. 2016. The brain imaging data structure, a format for organizing and describing outputs of neuroimaging experiments. *Scientific Data* 3. https://doi.org/10.1038/sdata.2016.44.

Greshake, Bastian, Philipp E. Bayer, Helge Rausch, and Julia Reda. 2014. openSNP – A crowdsourced web resource for personal genomics. *PLoS One* 9 (3): e89204. https://doi.org/10.1371/journal.pone.0089204.

Hackman, Daniel, and Farah Martha. 2008. Socioeconomic status and the developing brain. *Trends in Cognitive Science* 2009 Feb; 13 (2): 65–73. https://doi.org/10.1016/j.tics.2008.11.003.

Hackman, D.A., M.J. Farah, and M.J. Meaney. 2010. Socioeconomic status and the brain: Mechanistic insights from human and animal research. *Nature Reviews* 11: 651–659.

Haeusermann, Tobias, Bastian Greshake, Alessandro Blasimme, Darja Irdam, Martin Richards, and Effy Vayena. 2017. Open sharing of genomic data: Who does it and why? *PLoS One* 12 (5): 1–15. https://doi.org/10.1371/journal.pone.0177158.

Hanisch, Carol. 1969. *The personal is political*. http://www.carolhanisch.org/CHwritings/PIP.html.

Henrich, Joseph, Steven J. Heine, and Ara Norenzayan. 2010. The weirdest people in the world? *Behavioral and Brain Sciences* 33 (2–3): 61–83. https://doi.org/10.1017/S0140525X0999152X.

Kohane, Isaac S. 2015. Ten things we have to do to achieve precision medicine. *Science* 349 (6243): 37–38. https://doi.org/10.1126/science.aab1328.

Kovalevskaya, Nadezda V., Charlotte Whicher, Timothy D. Richardson, Craig Smith, Jana Grajciarova, Xocas Cardama, José Moreira, Adrian Alexa, Amanda A. McMurray, and Fiona G.G. Nielsen. 2016. DNAdigest and Repositive: Connecting the world of genomic data. *PLoS Biology* 14 (3). https://doi.org/10.1371/journal.pbio.1002418.

Kredlow, Alexandra M., Suzanne L. Pineles, Sabra S. Inslicht, Marie France Marin, Mohammed R. Milad, Michael W. Otto, and Scott P. Orr. 2017. Assessment of skin conductance in African American and non-African American participants in studies of conditioned fear. *Psychophysiology* 54 (11): 1741–1754. https://doi.org/10.1111/psyp.12909.

Kummar, Shivaani, P. Mickey Williams, Chih-Jian Lih, Eric C. Polley, Alice P. Chen, Larry V. Rubinstein, Yingdong Zhao, Richard M. Simon, Barbara A. Conley, and James H. Doroshow. 2015. Application of molecular profiling in clinical trials for advanced metastatic cancers. *JNCI-Journal of the National Cancer Institute* 107 (4): djv003. https://doi.org/10.1093/jnci/djv003.

Liddell, Belinda J., and Laura Jobson. 2016. The impact of cultural differences in self-representation on the neural substrates of posttraumatic stress disorder. *European Journal of Psychotraumatology* 1: 1–13. https://doi.org/10.3402/ejpt.v7.30464.

Lu, Y.-F., David B. Goldstein, Misha Angrist, and Gianpiero Cavalleri. 2014. Personalized medicine and human genetic diversity. *Cold Spring Harbor Perspectives in Medicine* 4 (9): a008581. https://doi.org/10.1101/cshperspect.a008581.

Madan, Christopher R. 2017. Advances in studying brain morphology: The benefits of open-access data. *Frontiers in Human Neuroscience* 11. https://doi.org/10.3389/fnhum.2017.00405.

Mao, Qing, Serban Ciotlos, Rebecca Yu, Madeleine P. Zhang, Robert Chin Ball, Paolo Carnevali, Nina Barua, et al. 2016. The whole genome sequences and experimentally phased haplotypes of over 100 personal genomes. *GigaScience* 5 (1). https://doi.org/10.1186/s13742-016-0148-z.

Marigorta, Urko M., Arcadi Navarro, P.M. Visscher, M.A. Brown, M.I. McCarthy, J. Yang, L.A. Hindorff, et al. 2013. High trans-ethnic replicability of GWAS results implies common causal variants. *PLoS Genetics* 9 (6): e1003566. https://doi.org/10.1371/journal.pgen.1003566.

Marshall, Narcis A., Hilary A. Marusak, Kelsey J. Sala-Hamrick, Laura M. Crespo, Christine A. Rabinak, and Moriah E. Thomason. 2018. Socioeconomic disadvantage and altered corticostriatal circuitry in urban youth. *Human Brain Mapping* 39 (5): 1982–1994. https://doi.org/10.1002/hbm.23978.

Martínez, Karen G., José A. Franco-Chaves, Mohammed R. Milad, and Gregory J. Quirk. 2014. Ethnic differences in physiological responses to fear conditioned stimuli. *PLoS One* 9 (12). https://doi.org/10.1371/journal.pone.0114977.

McAllister, Bryant F. 2017. *Exponential growth of the AncestryDNA database*. 2017.

Moon, Hojin, Hongshik Ahn, Ralph L. Kodell, Songjoon Baek, Chien-ju Lin, and James J. Chen. 2007. Ensemble methods for classification of patients for personalized medicine with high-dimensional data. *Moon* 41: 197–207. https://doi.org/10.1016/j.artmed.2007.07.003.

Niso, Guiomar, Christine Rogers, Jeremy T. Moreau, Li Yuan Chen, Cecile Madjar, Samir Das, Elizabeth Bock, et al. 2016. OMEGA: The Open MEG Archive. *NeuroImage* 124: 1182–1187. https://doi.org/10.1016/j.neuroimage.2015.04.028.

Niso, Guiomar, Krzysztof J. Gorgolewski, Elizabeth Bock, Teon L. Brooks, Guillaume Flandin, Alexandre Gramfort, Richard N. Henson, et al. 2018. MEG-BIDS, the brain imaging data structure extended to magnetoencephalography. *Scientific Data* 5: 180110. https://doi.org/10.1038/sdata.2018.110.

Parker, Nadine, Angelita Pui-Yee Wong, Gabriel Leonard, Michel Perron, Bruce Pike, Louis Richer, Suzanne Veillette, Zdenka Pausova, and Tomas Paus. 2017. Income inequality, gene expression, and brain maturation during adolescence. *Scientific Reports* 7 (1): 7397. https://doi.org/10.1038/s41598-017-07735-2.

Pink, Daniel H. 2005. *Why the world is flat*. WIRED. https://www.wired.com/2005/05/friedman-2/.

Poldrack, Russell A., Deanna M. Barch, Jason P. Mitchell, Tor D. Wager, Anthony D. Wagner, Joseph T. Devlin, Chad Cumba, Oluwasanmi Koyejo, and Michael P. Milham. 2013. Toward open sharing of task-based fMRI data: The OpenfMRI project. *Frontiers in Neuroinformatics* 7. https://doi.org/10.3389/fninf.2013.00012.

Poline, Jean-Baptiste, Janis L. Breeze, Satrajit Ghosh, Krzysztof Gorgolewski, Yaroslav Halchenko, Michael Hanke, Christian Haselgrove, et al. 2012. Data sharing in neuroimaging research. *Frontiers in Neuroinformatics* 6 (9). https://doi.org/10.3389/fninf.2012.00009.

"Problems with 23andMe ancestry composition". 2015. http://koreanhistoricaldramas.com/23andme-ancestry-composition/.

Roberts, A.L., S.E. Gilman, J. Breslau, N. Breslau, and K.C. Koenen. 2011. Race/ethnic differences in exposure to traumatic events, development of post-traumatic stress disorder, and treatment-seeking for post-traumatic stress disorder in the United States. *Psychological Medicine* 41 (1): 71–83. https://doi.org/10.1017/S0033291710000401.

Smith, Richard. 2012. Stratified, personalised, or precision medicine. *Thebmjopinion*.

Tan, Cong, and Xiang Du. 2012. KRAS mutation testing in metastatic colorectal Cancer. *World Journal of Gastroenterology* 18 (37): 5171–5180. https://doi.org/10.3748/wjg.v18.i37.5171.

Tzovara, Athina, Christoph W. Korn, and Dominik R. Bach. 2018. Human Pavlovian fear conditioning conforms to probabilistic learning. *PLoS Computational Biology* 14 (8): e1006243. https://doi.org/10.1371/journal.pcbi.1006243.

"UK10K". 2018. https://www.uk10k.org/.

Vorhaus, Don. 2010. The past, present and future of DTC genetic testing regulation. *Genomics Law Report*.

Weissman, David G., Rand D. Conger, Richard W. Robins, Paul D. Hastings, and Amanda E. Guyer. 2018. Income change alters default mode network connectivity for adolescents in poverty. *Developmental Cognitive Neuroscience* 30: 93–99. https://doi.org/10.1016/j.dcn.2018.01.008.

Wetterstrand, L.A. 2018. *DNA sequencing costs, data from the NHGRI genome sequencing program*. https://www.genome.gov/sequencingcostsdata/.

Chapter 9
Personal Data Cooperatives – A New Data Governance Framework for Data Donations and Precision Health

Ernst Hafen

Abstract Personalized health research depends on aggregated sets of personal data from millions of people. Given that personal data can be copied, individuals are entitled to copies of their data and individuals are the ultimate aggregators of all their personal data, citizens are elevated to new roles at the center of health research and a novel personal data economy. There, citizens, not some multinational company, control the use of and benefit from the intellectual and economic value of these data. Here, I show that democratically controlled nonprofit personal data cooperatives provide a governance and trust framework for data sharing and data donation. They also provide a means of attaining improved precision health and a digital society in which socio-economic asymmetries can be balanced.

Keywords Personal data · Electronic health records · EHR · Data portability · Data protection regulation · Empowerment · Cooperatives · Common good · Public health · Precision medicine · Artificial intelligence

9.1 The Unique Features of Personal Data

Medicine is transitioning from a heuristic science that is relying on relatively small numbers of cases to an increasingly data driven science involving large numbers of cases. Much of the data relevant to health research and efficient healthcare are personal data. These include data stored in medical records, registry databases and increasingly personal data recorded by patients/citizens themselves with the sensors in their smartphones. The challenges in using these data for research and better healthcare span from issues such as data silos, interoperability, data accessibility and obtaining the consent of individuals to access and use their data. Before

E. Hafen (✉)
Institute of Molecular Systems Biology, ETH Zürich, Zürich, Switzerland

MIDATA Cooperative, Zürich, Switzerland
e-mail: ehafen@ethz.ch

J. Krutzinna, L. Floridi (eds.), *The Ethics of Medical Data Donation*,
Philosophical Studies Series 137, https://doi.org/10.1007/978-3-030-04363-6_9

addressing these issues and offering at least partial solutions, I would like to highlight three special features of personal data: (1) Personal data, like other data, once generated, can easily be copied at near zero marginal costs. The copies can be used for different purposes. Data are a non-rivalrous good. Therefore, it is difficult to talk about data ownership. The doctor is bound by law to keep medical records for 15 years. Patients in most countries, however, have the right to obtain a copy of their medical records. (2) Personal data, or copies thereof, are a new asset class (World Economic Forum 2011). They comprise one of the few assets that are fairly equally distributed among people. All humans are billionaires in genome data since their genomes contain a unique set of six billion base pairs of DNA. Likewise, people have similar numbers of heart beats, steps and they consume a similar number of meals and liters of water. It is clear that access to resources like food and data is currently not equally distributed around the world. However, the rapid spread of smartphones and broadband internet in Low and Middle Income Countries (LMICs) has the potential to change this in the near future. (3) Individuals are the ultimate aggregators of their data. Only they will be in a position to aggregate data from their medical records, their genome data, their shopping data and their smartphone data. This is of course under the provision that they can obtain a copy of all these data. A right that, as we will see, has been strengthened greatly by the European General Data Protection Regulation (GDPR) (De Hert et al. 2017). The fact that data can be copied, data are equally distributed amongst individuals and that each individual is the ultimate aggregator of the data, forms a basis for a new role for patients and healthy individuals at the center of health research, prevention and care.

9.2 The Need – Aggregated Datasets on Millions of People

The human genome can be compared with the operating system of a smartphone. A smartphone app interacts with the operating system and produces a certain effect (e.g. recording and visualizing one's daily steps). A drug interferes with the human operating system to elicit an effect (e.g. relief of pain). We may ask why it takes two weeks to develop a smartphone app at a cost of $ 20,000, whereas it takes 15 years and $ 2bn to develop a drug. Moreover, we can expect the app to work on all smartphones using the same operating system, while drugs only work less than 50 percent of the time (Chhibber et al. 2014). Of course, the reasons for this difference are manifold. Above all is the fact that the smartphone operating systems were engineered and are thus completely understood, whereas the human operating system is a product of evolution (i.e. random mutations and natural selection evolution). Another difference, however, is that the copies of the operating system on smartphones are identical, whereas the human genomes of individuals differ in 1/1000 base pairs. The effectivity of drugs in pairs of identical twins is significantly higher than in fraternal twins or unrelated people (Chhibber et al. 2014). To improve the odds of medicine we need to learn how differences in genomes in combination with differences in environmental and behavioral factors affect health, disease and the treatment of disease. In other words, we need to make correlations between genotypes (genome) and phenotypes (health status) for millions of people. This is only possible with the active participation of the individuals as the rightful data aggregators and data access controllers themselves.

9.3 The Opportunity – The Legal Right of Citizens to Obtain Copies of Their Personal Data and Their Willingness to Contribute These Data to Research

9.3.1 The European General Data Protection Regulation (GDPR) – Data Portability

The new European Data Protection Regulation (GDPR) specifies in Article 20 the right of citizens to data portability permitting them to obtain machine readable copies of all their personal data (De Hert et al. 2017). This includes data on social networks, shopping data, medical, education data and other data. Initially planned as a way to create competition among data collectors in much the same way mobile phone providers guarantee that one's smartphone number is portable when changing providers, it results in a true empowerment of citizens in a data-driven environment. While individuals have little secondary use for their mobile phone numbers, they can aggregate and use copies of their medical, shopping, genome and fitness data in a variety of different ways. For example, they can actively participate in research projects by making their aggregated data sets accessible or they can profit from personalized data analysis services via apps provided by companies.

9.3.2 The Willingness and the Right to Citizen Science

There is a great willingness of people to actively participate and contribute to scientific research. This is evident from the millions of people who contribute their time, knowledge and data to citizen science platforms such as Zooniverse.org. On this platform, people help to annotate galaxies or wild-life in webcam images from the Serengeti, transcribe weather reports from old ship log books for occanic climate information and annotate histological sections for the existence of cancer cells. Increasingly, people also contribute to science not only as data scientists as in the above examples but also by directly collecting and contributing their own data to scientific projects. For example, the large majority of patients consent to using their medical data for medical research. At the university hospital in Lausanne a recent study showed that over 80 percent of the cancer patients provide a general consent for using their data including genome data for research (Mooser and Currat 2014). The willingness to contribute personal data to research is by no means limited to patients. Surveys with university students or elderly people who attend university programs for the elderly showed that roughly 60 percent would order a direct to consumer genetic test. The ability to support scientific research was mentioned by more people than to find out more about one's own genetic health risks (Vayena et al. 2014). Millions of citizens have even given their genome information to commercial companies such as 23andme.com or ancestry.com, even though they had to agree that their data is used commercially for the benefit of the companies' shareholders. Giving citizens the right to aggregate and control sharing of their personal data empowers them to become active participants in science (Vayena and Tasioulas 2016). In doing so, health relevant data collected continuously with smartphone sensors can be combined with medical and other data. The active participation in research projects also provides an excellent means to improve the scientific literacy of citizens and patients.

9.4 The Challenge

Smartphones have been available for more than 10 years and medical records also have existed, at least in some countries, in digital forms for even longer. Why then have citizens and patients not taken a more active role in managing their personal data and contributing to research? The reasons lie at least in part in the dynamics of the nascent personal data economy. Internet and social media companies, as well as app providers, provide their services for free in exchange for personal data. Because of the ease of use we have gotten used to paying for digital services with our personal data. These data fuel a nascent and rapidly growing personal data economy that is largely controlled by large multinational companies and data brokers. The value lies in the aggregation of these different data types for the purpose of digital and personalized advertising (Lanier 2010). As the recent case of Cambridge Analytica and Facebook shows, these data are increasingly also used for more subtle psychological manipulation including influencing political voting behavior (Dehaye 2017). Moreover, the companies controlling the largest amounts of data will have the best resource to train their artificial intelligence algorithms, thereby further increasing the socio-economic asymmetry between individuals all over the world and a few multinational companies (Haynes and Nguyen 2013; Lee 2017).

In the case of medical records, these are often locked in incompatible data silos in hospitals and the private practices of physicians. Even in countries where electronic health records (EHR) have been established, patients can access the records and make them accessible to other healthcare providers only for the primary use of the data, i.e. healthcare. There are few options to actively decide on the secondary use of these personal data for medical research or other data services. In order to aggregate medical and other health-related data under the control of the individual, a new governance framework that provides trust and empowerment for citizens/patients to aggregate and actively manage the access to their data is needed.

9.5 The Solution – Data Cooperatives and Personal Data, a Perfect Match

We posit that citizen-owned nonprofit data cooperatives provide the basis for a democratically controlled and fair personal data ecosystem from which society at large will profit. Democratic governance and self-help are part of the DNA of cooperatives and this sets them apart from other organizational forms including foundation and shareholder-controlled companies. The match between cooperative governance and personal data control rests on the three unique features of personal data.

First, data can be copied and individuals possess the right to obtain a digital copy of all their personal data according to the data portability article of the EU GDPR. This offers the possibility for a new parallel personal data ecosystem under the control of the citizens without directly interfering with the current personal data economy. Second, the fact that all people have similar amounts of personal data aligns well with the democratic one-member-one-vote governance of cooperatives. Third, the fact that individuals are the ultimate aggregators of their personal data offers the opportunity for entirely new data services, artificial intelligence and research on different data types that hitherto have been locked in different silos or whose access without the consent of the data subject is protected.

Data cooperatives operate a secure IT platform on which individuals can store, manage and control access to all their data copies. Much like the case of financial bank accounts, individual data account holders are in complete control over the use of their data. In contrast to most of the current banking software where administrators have access to customer data, however, in the personal data platform each record is encrypted and only the account holder has the key. Therefore, neither the administrator of the IT platform nor the management of the cooperative has access to the data. Account holders can become members of the cooperative and in this way also participate in the democratic governance of the cooperative. Their duties include the election of the board of the cooperative and to vote on how proceeds are invested (Hafen et al. 2014).

9.5.1 *Data Cooperatives, Business Model, Non-profit, Financial Incentives*

Data cooperatives act as the fiduciary of their respective account holders' data. When individuals make part or all their data accessible for academic or pharmaceutical research or for data services from other companies, the management of the cooperative negotiates access to these data with the researchers, pharmaceutical or data companies. It ensures that data access is fair. For example, data accessed by a data company providing a mobile app must not be sold to third parties, as is the case currently with all the "free" apps in the app stores. For research projects and clinical trials the cooperative ensures that the results generated with these personal data will be published irrespective of whether the results are positive or negative, and that copies of the data generated during the project will be returned to the individuals' accounts. It will also negotiate a fair price for data access by third parties. This can be a fee on mobile apps running on its platform, or for the recruitment of patients for clinical trials.

Will this cooperative model be profitable? The personal data economy, also called the digital identity economy, with the currently freely accessible data via social media, free apps and internet access is projected to reach a market volume of € 1 billion in 2020 in Europe (The Boston Consulting Group 2012). This figure does not include medical data, access to which is restricted by data protection laws. Combining these different data types under the control of the individuals will generate a vastly larger market value of which data cooperatives will obtain a significant share. By acting as the fiduciary of people's data and their decisions as to who and for what purpose their data can be accessed, data cooperatives negotiate the terms for data access with industrial partners, including pharmaceutical companies and data companies. The revenues generated from data access and also from the recruitment of consenting participants for clinical trials will be used to maintain and develop the platform, regular security checks and data services on the platform. Moreover, members of the cooperative will be able to vote on which research funds or data services revenues will be objects for investment. The nonprofit character of the data cooperative model specifies that these financial benefits will go back to society and not to the individuals who make their data accessible. There are two arguments for this statement, which at first glance may appear somewhat counterintuitive. First, although the aggregated data set of an individual is more valuable than the partial aggregates that companies and institutions possess of the same individual, the societal, intellectual and economic value lies not in the data set of a single individual but in those of all the participating individuals. We argue that this value should be returned to society at large. A distribution of dividends to members of the cooperative would be unfair, since many account holders may not want to become members and would therefore not profit from these dividends. Second, offering financial incentives for data sharing corrupts the motivation for sharing in much the same way blood donations work better without financial incentives (Sandel 2012).

9.5.2 Challenges to the Cooperative Model

Even though in general financial cooperatives fared better in the financial crisis than shareholder-controlled companies, there are plenty of reports about the failure of cooperatives (Birchall 2013). The establishment of personal data cooperatives faces two main challenges. First, establishing a truly participatory democratic governance with large numbers of members requires new tools such as liquid democracy, also called delegative or proxy democracy (Rutt 2018). Second, a major challenge for cooperatives is the initial financing. Even though data cooperatives will be hugely profitable with millions of account holders actively sharing data, establishing the platform, the initial services that provide a benefit for the users and the legal framework for the cooperative and data governance are challenging. In contrast to shareholder-controlled companies, cooperatives cannot give equity to financial investors, since they are owned by their respective members. Thus, cooperatives require initial financial support from foundations, from philanthropists and through research grants. Crowd financing is an obvious option but that would also require some tangible short term benefits for it to succeed.

9.5.3 Example: MIDATA Data Cooperative

The MIDATA cooperative is a first example of a data cooperative that shows how data can be used for the common good, while at the same time ensuring the citizens' sovereignty over their personal data. Founded in 2015, the non-profit cooperative operates a data platform, acts as a trustee for data collection and guarantees the sovereignty of citizens over the use of their data. The citizens actively contribute to research as users of the platform by providing access to data sets and as cooperative members to control and develop the cooperative. Currently, the Swiss MIDATA cooperative accepts only residents of Switzerland. With partners in Germany, Belgium, the Netherlands and the United Kingdom, we are setting up MIDATA cooperatives in these countries.

The articles of association of the cooperative define its nature as a non-profit organization and enshrine the sovereignty of users over their data and its use (including use in anonymized form). An internal cooperative data ethics review board, whose members are elected by the general assembly, controls the ethical quality of the services and related projects. Members and non-members of the cooperative can open an account and possess the same rights on the platform. Members participate also in the governance of the platform.

9.5.4 The Data Platform and Governance Form the Core of a New Innovation Ecosystem

The data platform used by MIDATA is being developed by ETH Zürich and the Bern University of Applied Sciences. It allows citizens to collect their health data and to freely decide on the use of that data in research projects. They can thus play an active role in medical research as "citizen scientists".

The platform model allows the separation of the IT platform (data storage, access and consent management) from the data applications (mobile applications) and thus enables an open innovation ecosystem. Users will have access to various data services and can decide to participate in research projects. Start-ups, IT service providers and research groups can offer mobile apps on the platform, for example, health apps or apps for the management of chronic diseases.

The IT platform is operational and is currently being used in several data science projects. In one project, patients after a gastric bypass operation record their condition, fitness and weight at home and share the data with the attending physician at the Bern University Hospital. In another project at the Zürich University Hospital, patients suffering from multiple sclerosis are testing the effect of treatments using a tablet app that assesses their cognitive and motor status. In the allyscience.ch project, people suffering from hay fever record their symptoms and contribute to a Swiss-wide allergy map in relation to pollen data provided by Meteo Swiss. More than 8,000 people have downloaded the AllyScience App and actively contribute as citizen scientists to this project.

9.6 Data Cooperatives and Data Donations

In the Middle Ages, feudal lords argued that they could not pay their serfs money for their work since the serfs could not handle the responsibility and would immediately spend it on drink and women. Today, most people in high income countries have a bank account and decide how to invest or spend their money. This forms the basis of our current economy and the globally improved standards of living. Inheritance of financial assets is also clearly regulated. In 5–10 years, people will possess their own data bank account and decide to whom and for what purpose they will provide access to their data. As in the case of banks today, there will be different business models for such data banks. Some may offer citizens financial incentives and maximize the profits for shareholders, others will be non-profit cooperatives whose revenues will be invested for the common good. Personal data is much more personal than money. Trust will be the most essential factor in generating a citizen-controlled personal data economy. In such a trusted environment people will become active contributors and actors in the digital society. By learning the benefit of data sharing for public health and as well as their own health and wellbeing they will be prepared do donate their data post mortem for the common good.

Even though the digital revolution threatens to further increase the global digital dependence of individuals from data and AI service providing companies and augment the socio-economic asymmetries, it also offers a new avenue out of this dependency. With their unique personal data assets, individuals can help to democratize the personal data economy and contribute to John Rawls' vision of the most just form of society, a property-owning democracy in which people possess not only a political but also an economic vote (Rawls 2009). With their personal data, citizens all over the world now possess an equally distributed economic value that in combination with a cooperative governance as outlined above could contribute to such just societies globally.

References

Birchall, J. 2013. *Resilience in a Downturn: The Power of Financial Cooperatives*. Geneva: ILO.

Chhibber, A., D.L. Kroetz, K.G. Tantisira, et al. 2014. Genomic architecture of pharmacological efficacy and adverse events. *Pharmacogenomics* 15 (16): 2025–2048. https://doi.org/10.2217/pgs.14.144.

De Hert, P., V. Papakonstantinou, G. Malgieri, L. Beslay, and I. Sanchez. 2017. The right to data portability in the GDPR: Towards user-centric interoperability of digital services. *Computer Law & Security Review: The International Journal of Technology Law and Practice* 34 (2): 1–11. https://doi.org/10.1016/j.clsr.2017.10.003.

Dehaye, P.O. 2017. *Cambridge Analytica and Facebook data*. Medium. Retrieved May 23, 2017.

Hafen, E., D. Kossmann, and A. Brand. 2014. Health data cooperatives – Citizen empowerment. *Methods of Information in Medicine* 53 (2): 82–86. https://doi.org/10.3414/ME13-02-0051.

Haynes, P., and C.M.-H. Nguyen. 2013. Rebalancing socioeconomic asymmetry in a data-driven economy. In *The global information technology report*, ed. B. Bilbao-Osorio, S. Dutta, and B. Lanvin, 67–72. Geneva: World Economic Forum.

Lanier, J. 2010. *You are not a gadget*. Vintage.

Lee, K. Opinion|The real threat of artificial intelligence. June 2017. https://www.nytimes.com/2017/06/24/opinion/sunday/artificial-intelligence-economic-inequality.html.

Mooser, V., and C. Currat. 2014. The Lausanne Institutional Biobank: A new resource to catalyse research in personalised medicine and pharmaceutical sciences. *Swiss Medical Weekly* 144: w14033. https://doi.org/10.4414/smw.2014.14033.

Rawls, J.A. 2009. *Theory of justice*. Cambridge, MA: Harvard University Press.

Rutt, J. 2018. *An introduction into liquid democracy*. Medium. https://medium.com/@memetic007/liquid-democracy-9cf7a4cb7f. Accessed 25 Aug 2018.

Sandel, M.J. 2012. *Sandel: What money can't buy: The moral limits of markets – Google scholar*.

The Boston Consulting Group. 2012. *The value of our digital identity*, 1–65. http://www.liberty-global.com/PDF/public-policy/The-Value-of-Our-Digital-Identity.pdf.

Vayena, E., and J. Tasioulas. 2016. The dynamics of big data and human rights: The case of scientific research. *Philosophical Transactions of The Royal Society A Mathematical Physical and Engineering Sciences* 374 (2083): 20160129. https://doi.org/10.1098/rsta.2016.0129.

Vayena, E., C. Ineichen, E. Stoupka, and E. Hafen. 2014. Playing a part in research? University students' attitudes to direct-to-consumer genomics. *Public Health Genomics* 17 (3): 158–168. https://doi.org/10.1159/000360257.

World Economic Forum. 2011. *Personal data: The emergence of a new asset class*, 1–40. World Economic Forum.

Chapter 10
Defining Data Donation After Death: Metadata, Families, Directives, Guardians and the Route to Big Consent

David M. Shaw

Abstract This chapter explores what we actually mean by data donation after death, and what different types of data donation metadata are involved in the process. It then provides an analysis of the ethical ramifications of each of these different types of data, outlines the concepts of data advance directives and data donation guardians as one way of dealing with these issues, and considers alternative governance mechanisms. The degree of control given to the first data donors may need to be high in order to maintain trust, but over time attitudes may evolve towards everyone giving "big consent" to data donation.

Keywords Data donation after death · Ethics · Big consent · Posthumous data donation · Advance directives · Data guardians

10.1 Introduction

With the advent of the General Data Protection Regulation (GDPR) (EU 2016) and the Cambridge Analytica scandal (Schenble et al. 2018), public awareness of the issues surrounding data governance has never been higher. The GDPR aims to better protect citizens' data rights, while also enabling research and other important activities to proceed under certain conditions. In this context, the very idea of data donation might seem naïve; who would want to donate sensitive data, when 'donation' implies an unconditional gift for the recipient to dispose of as he or she pleases? Data donation after death might be seen as more attractive because the donor can no longer be directly affected by (mis-)use of data, but dead people also cannot raise concerns about any such misuse. In this chapter, I explore what is actually meant by

D. M. Shaw (✉)
Institute for Biomedical Ethics, University of Basel, Basel, Switzerland

Care and Public Health Research Institute, Maastricht University, Maastricht, The Netherlands
e-mail: david.shaw@unibas.ch

J. Krutzinna, L. Floridi (eds.), *The Ethics of Medical Data Donation*, Philosophical Studies Series 137, https://doi.org/10.1007/978-3-030-04363-6_10

"data donation after death" (DDD), and analyse the advantages and disadvantages of various potential governance mechanisms.

I begin by setting out what is meant by DDD in general terms, before illustrating the issues by means of comparison with the established practice of posthumous organ donation. I then explain and analyse the ethical ramifications of the five main types of data donation metadata: whether the related item of medical data can be shared at all, who else is affected by the data, with whom the data can be shared, in what form the data can be shared, and who has authority to change any of the previous four 'settings'. I then sketch the outlines of a potential system whereby donors could impose certain conditions on their data donations. I conclude by considering alternative forms of governance, including ethical oversight of unconditional DDD.

10.2 Defining Data Donation After Death

When people die they leave lots of data behind. This includes financial data, data on social media, governmental and tax data, and personally owned data including (for example) electronic movies and songs, and in some cases creative data such as songs and literary compositions. But for the purposes of this paper, I focus on clinical data and medical research data. When a patient dies he leaves behind not only a medical record, but also any data used in research projects. Despite the person's departure, this data remains an immensely powerful resource, particularly if it can be combined with other datasets. (Indeed, in many cases the nature of the person's departure will also be a relevant data point, if disease linked.) But how can this data be donated? The simplest way to explain DDD is to use organ donation as an example. There are many parallels but also some dissimilarities between DDD and deceased donation of organs (DDO) (Shaw et al. 2015). Both the similarities and the differences are helpful in terms of determining how we should think about DDD and how it should be governed.

In DDO, organs are donated after one's death and distributed among one or more recipients. Consent can come from the donor, via the organ donor register, or from a family member, where there is no record of consent. In 'opt-out' jurisdictions consent can also be 'deemed' or presumed if there is no record of objection. It is important to note that, despite having no legal right to do so, family members often overrule donation even when there is evidence of consent (NHSBT 2017) – this may also be relevant to data donation. DDO is essentially unconditional; no terms can be imposed on who or what type of person can receive the organs (to avoid any discriminatory criteria being imposed), and there are no guarantees that any organs will be transplanted at all. However, donors can stipulate which organs they want to donate; most donors donate all organs, but some choose not to donate specific organs such as the eyes, or the heart.

Should DDD be approached in the same way as DDO? In both cases the patient is dead, and if the language of donation is being used then presumably consent must be given – or at least presumed. Should data donors be able to stipulate who they donate to, or what types of data? To answer these questions and others we first need to consider the various types of data donation metadata.

10.3 Data Donation Metadata

For each item of data in a person's medical record, or associated research data, there could be several items of metadata indicating that donor's preferences regarding how their data should be used, and setting the terms of their donation. Specifically, each piece of data could(at least) five key data concerning it: whether it can be shared at all; who (if anyone) else it concerns; who it can be shared with; what form it can be shared in; and who (if anyone) needs to give consent for any other type of sharing (see Box 10.1). Each of these must be examined in turn.

First, a person might not want some categories of data to be shared at all. This is most likely to be the case for sensitive sexual health data, or genetic data, which could yield paternity information relevant to other family members. If a category of data is excluded from sharing with anyone, there need be no data regarding it in the second, third or fourth categories of metadata, though there should also be a corresponding entry for the fifth type, as a representative might be empowered to give future consent for this type of data to be shared.

Box 10.1: Data Donation Metadata
Whether it can be shared
Who (if anyone) else it concerns
Who it can be shared with
What form it can be shared in
Who needs to give consent for any other type of sharing

Second, medical data can concern not only the patient to whom it pertains directly, but also his or her family. Though it can also concern other types of medical data, this is particularly true of genetic data. A well-meaning data donor might not consider the fact that if he makes an unconditional donation, it could reveal that his son or daughter also has (or is likely to have) a particular genetic condition, with potential ramifications for privacy and insurance. Should people be able to donate their genetic data when they die? It is "theirs" but it also concerns others, even if this is only in terms of probabilities rather than certainties in many cases, due to genetic data often yielding no definitive answer. In organ donation, families often refuse to give consent to donation or overrule consent because they are upset by the idea of losing 'more' of their relative. Should families have a right to veto data donation, at least in terms of genetic data? In organ donation there is normally little ethical basis for a genuine overrule of what the patient wanted (UKDEC 2016), but given that genetic information can apply to other family members, there are potentially more solid grounds for legitimate objection. Another possibility would be for the rights of families to be protected by some oversight mechanism such as an ethics committee, but this might be impractical (see next section). (As noted above, non-genetic health information can also yield information on family members; for instance, if a deceased patient had a history of heart disease, this information might be of use to insurers. However, genetic information can reveal definitively whether offspring have or do not have a particular condition, and thus might be regarded as more sensitive.)

Third, people might be happy to donate their medical data posthumously, but not without imposing conditions on who can access that data. For example, evidence from a large UK study suggests that (living) citizens are generally happy to share their data with the National Health Service and associated researchers, rather less happy to share data with university researchers, and downright unhappy to share data with private companies such as the large pharmaceutical ones (Wellcome 2013). People might be more relaxed about sharing data posthumously, but they might also want to exert some degree of control over the potential recipients of their data. If people are denied this control, they might simply refuse to donate any data at all; this was one of the unfortunate features of the ill-fated care.data initiative in England, where patients only had a binary option: either all their data was shared, or none of it at all (Shaw 2014). However, one problem with limiting the recipients of data in this way is that industry often collaborates with the National Health Service (NHS), and vice versa. Ultimately, it transpired that even this simple binary option was too complex; those who opted out had their data shared anyway, indicating the lack of seriousness accorded to data consent in the NHS (Ramesh 2015).

Fourth, data can be shared in four main forms: fully identifiable, de-identified, pseudonymised and fully anonymised. Fully identifiable data reveals a donor's name, date of birth, address, demographics and full medical history. Anonymised data reveals only the medical history, with no location or other data revealed. De-identified data removes personal and demographic information. Pseudonymised information is anonymized data that can be re-linked to patient identifiers using an encoded key (Ohmann et al. 2017). People might be reluctant to share the first of these, but be more content with sharing of pseudonymised data. Generally, people are more comfortable sharing anonymised data as it cannot be linked back to them (Wellcome 2013), but they might be more comfortable sharing de-identified or fully identifiable data in the case of DDD because there is (even) less risk of any adverse consequences to donors who are dead; however, the potential risk to surviving family members remains. It is important to note that in the era of big data and machine learning, de-identified and even anonymised data could potentially be linked with other datasets and thus to specific donors, so the distinctions between these four forms of data are being eroded (Schneble et al. 2018).

Fifth, donors might want to grant authority to a trusted person or organisation to give consent to other future uses of the donated data. This might be prudent because once a person is dead, she can obviously no longer be involved in any such decisions, and circumstances might mean that she would have wanted to change something were she not dead. By donating, donors give consent to any uses of his or her data within the terms set in their metadata (perhaps subject to further safeguards – see next section). The nominated person would not be required to give consent to all uses of data, but would be approached where a project outwith the scope of the donor's metadata settings wanted to use data.

Finally, it is also important to bear in mind that all of these metadata are interlinked. For example, a person might be happy to share anonymised general medical data with everyone, but restrict use of identifiable medical data and any genetic data to the NHS. They might also be willing to grant authority for a trusted person or organisation to change their preferences for some types of data, but not for all.

10.4 Data Advance Directives

What is the best way to record one's data donation preference metadata? I have previously suggested a data donor card similar to an organ donor card (Shaw et al. 2015) but an instrument for setting preferences in advance already exists in medicine: the advance directive. A data advance directive (DAD) would record all the relevant information mentioned in the previous section, setting the defaults for use of that donor's data.

Setting up a DAD would be a one-time procedure, thought it could of course be altered at any point up to a person's death. Users would be guided through setting up each metadata preference via a decision tree for ease of use. From the initial question - something like "would you like to share your data after death to help researchers?" - questions would probably best be focused on categories of medical and research data, with each group of data having its own metadata preferences as set out above. The second category, regarding who else data concerns, would not be available as a preference but would be set by system guardians. Depending on the jurisdiction, it is possible that genetic data could be shared only with the permission of family members. Thus for each type of data, the user could determine whether to share it at all, and if so (and dependent on whether it also concerns family members) who it can be shared with, in what form, and whether the terms they set for the use of their data can be altered in future by a designated person.

10.5 Posthumous Data Guardians

As stated above, DADs will go a long way towards governing deceased persons' data responsibly. But the final part of setting up a DAD should be to nominate a survivor who can be consulted above any exceptions to the set terms, or potentially to change them permanently. These Posthumous Data Guardians (PDGs) would perform an important backup role, made all the more significant by ongoing rapid advances in data handling techniques. For example, it might be that in 10 years the category of "de-identified" data will disappear entirely, necessitating a change in DAD preferences to reflect what that user would probably have wanted to do in such circumstances. In addition, some people might not want to set up a DAD, preferring to delegate responsibility for posthumous use of their data to a surrogate. This could be implemented as an option, but would require this person to be contacted for each potential data useage, which would really mean that the data was not donated at all.

10.6 Objections

The combination of DADs and PDGs offers a flexible way for donors to set their preferences and safeguard their (and their families') interests after they die. The main objection to the metadata, DAD and PDG proposal detailed above is that donation should be unconditional, for two main reasons: enabling preference-setting would be against the spirit of donation, and that it would be much more practical to simply have donation of all data.

Is enabling some preferences to be set against the spirit of donation? As already mentioned, organ donors can choose which organs to donate. When people die they can allocate their financial reserves and possessions to wherever they want. Data is highly personal, and if people want to set limits on its use after they are dead, there must be a strong argument against letting them do so – not least because removing the ability to set preferences will push people towards refusing entirely to donate their data.

The second argument about practicality has more force. The more preferences that can be set, the more complicated it is for researchers to combine datasets and some patients' data might be rendered entirely inaccessible. But as stated above, it might be even less practical to alienate donors by not enabling preference-setting.

One other possibility in addition to DADs and PDGs would be to enable donors to set a "data death date" beyond which their data can no longer be used – for example, at 50 years after death. This would set a final boundary on the use of donated data, but it is not obvious that many would find this option attractive. Why share data after your death, but only for a limited period? One potential reason would be that the the risk of unanticipated types of research using ones' data might increase over time, and a time-limit on its use would decrease this risk. However, after decades have passed, a donor's data could have been aggregated and imbedded in thousands of different analyses, and stopping use of it might be highly impractical even if there was a good reason for allowing donors to set such an expiry date. Allowing control so far beyond the grave would also constrain the public benefits flowing from the initial donation.

10.7 Other Governance Mechanisms

Taken together, even for just one person, the amount of data involved in DDD means that we are essentially talking about big data, and hence not simply data donation but actually 'big data donation'. That in turn means that what is needed is big data protection; protection not only of the data concerning an individual, but also of the potential benefit to the public of big data research (Shaw 2017). DAD would be one way of providing this. But if we were to reject detailed preference-setting as set out above, and aim to embrace a less controlling, more openly altruistic model of data donation, what alternative governance mechanisms exist?

One option would be for donation to be regarded as broad consent to future research, subject to future research ethics committee (REC) review. This option already exists outwith the context of donation; in many consent forms, participants can not only agree to take part in a given study, but also for their data or samples to be used in any future study, subject to REC review. This model could work, but suffers from two main drawbacks. First, giving certain limited data and perhaps one or two biological samples is rather different from donating all the medical data ever generated about yourself. Donating unconditionally all your medical and genetic information and trusting RECs to always approve only 'safe' projects may be asking too much of potential donors, particularly in the coming era of ethics review equivalency, where some have suggested that additional REC review may not be required when new countries start participating in a study. Second, any unconditional donation will last essentially forever. Setting preferences and nominating a guardian at least offers some degree of control over future use of data.

Another alternative would be a move towards not research ethics committees, but research ethics communities, where it is assumed that everyone will contribute their data both while living and once dead in order to show solidarity with and benefit their community (Shaw 2017). This would be the ideal solution; a world in which everyone unconditionally donates their data. But it may be unrealistic to try to step straight to such a world. The combination of DADs and PDGs in DDD is a safe first step towards encouraging people to trust researchers with their data. Following this, the use of this preference scheme could be extended to data donation whilst alive, before trialling unconditional donation after death and ultimately a community where everyone shares their health data all the time. Notably, any such research ethics community would at a stroke solve the issue of family data sharing – if all family members share data routinely through solidarity, no concerns about genetic information need remain.

However, families remain an issue for unconditional data donation in the present day. While many, or even most relatives might be happy for their family members to donate genetic and other data when they die, others might not, and it is difficult to see how someone can donate data that is not entirely theirs, as it is thus not entirely in their gift. The fact that genetic data concerns not only ourselves but also our family members may be a significant barrier to the very concept of data donation.

It might be objected that family members have no say in whether we share our genetic or other medical data while we are alive; why, then, should they have a say when we are dead? It is true that each living person is free to share any personal medical information that he or she pleases with researchers, without constraint by any relatives. However, this is because a living person has certain rights regarding his or her data, even if it affects their family members. Once that person is dead, the only people that can be directly affected by use of that data are the deceased's family members, and the balance of control should shift accordingly – not entirely to the family, but towards shared control over the data.

For this reason it might be better to think in terms of dual consent to data donation after death, rather than simple data donation after death. A person can consent to donation, and this donation can proceed only if potentially affected family members also consent. A data donor can consent to use of his or her data, but cannot consent regarding data that also concerns family members. Therefore, a type of dual consent might be required for full data donation after death. This is unfortunate, but the path towards full data sharing will not be paved with good intentions if families are not on board with the first models of data donation. Ultimately, as stated above, a move towards a research ethics community, where every one is happy to give not specific or narrow, nor broad, nor general but 'big consent' to all use of all 'their' big data without restrictions, whether or not it concerns their family members.

10.8 Conclusion

In this paper, I have suggested that, while DDD could ultimately be unconditional, any such scheme must begin by allowing donors to set certain preferences. Encouraging potential donors to create data advance directives is the first step towards a world in which data sharing for the common good is 'automatic for the people', both in the sense of being a common good, but also being second nature. The route to big consent must begin with dual consent to data donation.

References

General Data Protection Regulation (GDPR) (EU) 2016/679.

National Health Service Blood and Transplant. 2017. *National potential donor audit.*

Ohmann, C., R. Banzi, S. Canham, et al. 2017. Sharing and reuse of individual participant data from clinical trials: Principles and recommendations. *BMJ Open* 7: e018647. https://doi.org/10.1136/bmjopen-2017-018647.

Ramesh, R. 2015. NHS disregards patient requests to opt out of sharing medical records. *The Guardian*, 22nd January 2015. https://www.theguardian.com/society/2015/jan/22/nhs-disregards-patients-requests-sharing-medical-records. Accessed 21 Aug 2018.

Schneble, C.O., Elger, B.S., and Shaw, D. 2018. *The Cambridge Analytica affair and Internet-mediated research*, EMBO reports 2018. Online early. https://doi.org/10.15252/embr.201846579.

Shaw, D. 2014. Care. data, consent and confidentiality. *Lancet* 383: 1205.

———. 2017. Ethics review equivalency, moral jurisdiction and research ethics communities. *Medicine and Law* 36: 51–59 big data protection.

Shaw, D., J. Gross, and T. Erren. 2015. Data donation after death. *EMBO Reports* 17: 14–17. https://doi.org/10.15252/embr.201541802.

UK Donation Ethics Committee (UKDEC). 2016. *Involving the family in deceased organ donation: A discussion paper*. Academy of Medical Royal Colleges.

Wellcome Trust. 2013. Summary report of qualitative research into public attitudes to personal data and linking personal data, July. Available at: http://www.wellcome.ac.uk/About-us/Publications/Reports/Publicengagement/WTP053206.htm.

Part IV
An Ethical Code for Posthumous Medical Data Donation

Chapter 11
Enabling Posthumous Medical Data Donation: A Plea for the Ethical Utilisation of Personal Health Data

Jenny Krutzinna, Mariarosaria Taddeo, and Luciano Floridi

Abstract This article argues that personal medical data should be made available for scientific research, by enabling and encouraging individuals to donate their medical records once deceased, in a way similar to how they can already donate organs or bodies. This research is part of a project on posthumous medical data donation (PMDD) developed by the Digital Ethics Lab at the Oxford Internet Institute. Ten arguments are provided to support the need to foster posthumous medical data donation. Two major risks are also identified—harm to others, and lack of control over the use of data—which could follow from unregulated donation of medical data. The argument that record-based medical research should proceed without the need to ask for informed consent is rejected, and it instead a voluntary and participatory approach to using personal medical data should be followed. The analysis concludes by stressing the need to develop an ethical code for data donation to minimise the risks providing five foundational principles for ethical medical data donation; and suggesting a draft for such a code.

Keywords Data donation · Medical data ethics · Ethical code · Data philanthropy

J. Krutzinna (✉)
Department of Administration and Organization Theory, University of Bergen, Bergen, Norway
e-mail: jenny.krutzinna@uib.no

M. Taddeo · L. Floridi
Oxford Internet Institute, University of Oxford, Oxford, UK

The Alan Turing Institute, London, UK
e-mail: mariarosaria.taddeo@oii.ox.ac.uk; luciano.floridi@oii.ox.ac.uk

J. Krutzinna, L. Floridi (eds.), *The Ethics of Medical Data Donation*, Philosophical Studies Series 137, https://doi.org/10.1007/978-3-030-04363-6_11

11.1 Introduction

Numerous health conditions affecting large parts of the population remain under-researched. The consequence is that preventative measures, treatments and/or cures are lacking. Some of these illnesses, such as Alzheimer's dementia or Parkinson's disease, have devastating effects on their sufferers, and currently lack adequate treatment. While some progress has been made in discovering genetic or biological markers to identify people at greater risk of contracting certain diseases, little is known about the interpersonal differences that make someone a sufferer while sparing others with identical markers. Identifying and understanding these underlying differences is hard partly because of a lack of relevant data. The data required for such scientific progress need to be wide and longitudinal, but this is difficult and costly to obtain within traditional clinical research studies. At the same time, some data that exist are currently unavailable to research due to the absence of an adequate framework to streamline the currently onerous access procedures. Although individuals can volunteer while alive their data to private corporations by accepting terms and conditions to this effect, it is not yet possible to give one's medical data (whether during life or after death), for research purposes to a public institution. Nor is there any regulatory or ethical framework in place to guide the donation process. In this article, we argue that this constitutes an unethical failure to utilise data that are of immense value and importance in the quest to improve public health and to promote the common good. The focus is on posthumous medical data donation (PMDD), which should be enabled as a matter of urgency by putting in place an ethical code of PMDD.

The article starts with an outline of what is meant by PMDD, followed by an explanation of the reasons for enabling PMDD. These consist of 10 arguments in favour of PMDD, as well as arguments against the alternative approach suggested by some researchers (e.g. Mann et al. 2016), namely the removal of the need for individual informed consent in Big Data health research. Comparing PMDD to other types of biomedical donations that already take place, we argue that the existing ethical frameworks from other donation schemes provide useful guidance, but do not suffice to ensure ethical PMDD. Therefore, we stress the need to define an ethical code specific to PMDD, and propose five foundational principles for such a code.

11.2 What Is Posthumous Medical Data Donation?

Posthumous medical data donation (PMDD) refers to the act of donating one's personal medical data after death. Medical data is meant to describe here data that are routinely collected in a health system, whenever individuals use health services, throughout their life. Such data hold enormous potential for medical research and for health and care improvements on a large scale. However, personal medical data

Table 11.1 Differences between data donation, sharing and philanthropy

	Data source	Dataset
Data donation	Deceased individual	Single dataset
Data sharing	Living individual, researcher	Single or multiple
Data philanthropy	Institutional	Multiple, large-scale

currently remain mostly inaccessible for researchers due to a lack of enabling regulation. Issues of consent, ownership, and privacy, among others, mean that upon death, an individual's data become 'locked in'. Depending on the jurisdiction, gaining access for research purposes is cumbersome, if possible at all (Shaw et al. 2015). An effective way to solve this problem is by making provisions for enabling the donation of one's own medical data after death. So far, the *donation* of medical data has received limited attention (Shaw et al. 2016).

PMDD is different from medical data *sharing*,[1] which happens while one is alive, and from medical data *philanthropy*, which describes the opening, to external access and use, by private companies and public organisations, of their data sets, for charitable purposes (Taddeo 2016).[2] Data sharing and philanthropy are important sources of medical information, but, as we shall argue in the rest of this article, posthumous medical data *donation* is motivated by different reasons, and is less risky and more easily achievable than either data sharing or data philanthropy (Table 11.1).

Other types of donation in the medical field are already very common. Indeed, a significant part of the medical system relies on donations to save lives, educate and teach the medical profession, and advance medical knowledge in general. Examples include blood, organ and tissue donations, gamete donations, stem cell and cord blood donations, as well as brain and body donations for research and educational purposes. It is even possible to donate one's body for commercial or artistic purposes, albeit controversially, for instance to the anatomist and inventor of plastination, Gunther von Hagens, and his (in)famous "Body Worlds" exhibition.[3]

Unlike these types of biomedical donation, the donation of medical *data* is conceptually problematic: a lack of materiality and the simultaneity of data pose a challenge to the notion that data can be "donated" in the conventional sense (Prainsack 2018). However, at least in the context of post-mortem donations, the use of 'donation' appears preferable to more general terms, like 'sharing', as the former rules out the possibility of a retraction of the data by the donor or of joint use with the donor.

When it comes to donating medical data, there are specific subsets of data that can currently be donated. One such example is genomic data (Haeusermann et al.

[1] It has been argued that data sharing is a misleading concept and should be abandoned: See "Why we should stop talking about data sharing", Barbara Prainsack, (2015), http://dnadigest.org/why-we-should-stop-talking-about-data-sharing/ (accessed July 20, 2018).

[2] Also see: "Data Philanthropy: Where Are We Now?" United Nations Global Pulse. https://www.unglobalpulse.org/data-philanthropy-where-are-we-now (accessed March 5, 2018).

[3] See https://bodyworlds.com/ (accessed November 5, 2018).

2017). For instance, the Personal Genome Project enables individuals to "donate" their full genome for research purposes.[4] Another example is data given during participation in medical research projects, studies, or clinical trials. However, the donation of a more comprehensive dataset, such as in the form of personal medical records (PMRs) has not been systematically enabled so far. The collection and use of medical data for research purposes has mostly been via the aforementioned patient surveys, clinical studies, and trials. As the type and number of patients recruited to these is rather limited, a vast amount of potential data is not included and remains unused. At the same time, the infrastructure of our health services is changing to enable—in theory—the wider sharing of data with health care professionals and researchers. For instance, through the electronic health records (EHRs) currently being introduced within NHS England, individuals can share their own records via a link. This still faces some challenges, partly due to different data formats and a lack of data system interoperability.[5] In addition, serious limitations of this approach relate to the quality of information and the fact that the data available in these EHRs tend to be incomplete, and vary from General Practitioner (GP) practice to GP practice, but these are predominantly practical obstacles that could easily be overcome (Floridi and Illari 2016).

The failure to utilise fully the health data available in PMRs, which often already exist in digitised form as EHRs, has a huge opportunity cost. It has a negative effect on medical research, given that an incredibly valuable resource remains untapped when its utilisation could lead to significant advances in medical knowledge. In times when public health is in desperate need of improvement and when many serious health conditions are poorly understood, this is unacceptable and, it is argued, unethical. It is crucial to enable individuals to donate their medical data and enable its use for research for the common good.

11.3 Why We Should Enable PMDD

In light of the potential benefit to be derived from the utilisation of PMRs for research purposes, some have suggested that obtaining informed consent from individuals is inappropriate for record-based research (Mann et al. 2016). This position emphasises the benefit for society at large, and maintains that because of a "duty to easy rescue"—i.e. that individuals are under a moral obligation to benefit others where there is no or minimal risk to themselves—one would be justified in bypassing, in this particular context, what is otherwise a fundamental principle in research ethics: informed consent. Indeed, the current legal rules in many Western jurisdictions

[4]The use of "donate" in the context of the PGP is based on the PGPs own description: See https://www.personalgenomes.org.uk/ (accessed July 20, 2018).

[5]An additional and often overlooked challenge lies in the fact that at least the textual passages of any medical records are likely to be the subject of copyright and would need to be released prior to any donation. However, practical solutions to such challenges could be found, for instance, by reaching an agreement with public health institutions, such as the NHS, on an organisational level.

allow for this type of research to proceed without such consent, but this article is concerned primarily with the *ethical* considerations relating to PMDD, and not with legal frameworks.

There is clearly some merit in reconsidering how informed consent operates in modern data- or record-based medical research, where in order to maximise utility, data often need to be repurposed in ways that could not have been anticipated at the time of data collection. Rather than negating a need for consent in such instances, however, we consider it ethically preferable to enable those individuals *already willing* to volunteer their data to do so, even if this may lead to an initial and perhaps unavoidable bias, but one which may also be acceptable in order to start the process.[6] Note that empirical research into patient attitudes suggests that they are many.[7] This approach will foster trust and encourage wider social acceptance of the collection and re-use of medical data. However, if such a fully voluntary approach does not yield sufficient participation, a move towards an alternative approach is conceivable, e.g. through an opt-out system or record-based research with less consent requirements attached. In addition, abandoning the informed consent requirement on the basis of an analogical reasoning in terms of rescue seems inappropriate, where no discernible individual is immediately saved or even treated. The long-term time horizon of most medical research projects also makes it rather unlikely that the patient data subjects will ever become beneficiaries of any research findings resulting directly from their own records. This is obviously impossible in the case of data of the deceased. Therefore, the idea of simply using the available data without first obtaining informed consent is dismissed, even where this would be within the current limits of the law. Instead, from an ethical perspective, PMDD should be enabled and encouraged as a fully voluntary action for the following ten reasons.

(1) It is unethical to frustrate the "*will-to-do-it*" without proper justification. Although no individual donor will receive a benefit at the point of donation, the ability to contribute to the advancement of medicine and act as a moral agent can provide a significant benefit during one's lifetime. Studies with organ, body, and brain donors show a strong desire to do *post-mortem good*, and suggest that medical data would be no different (Steinsbekk et al. 2013). Indeed, the Personal Genome Project and patient networks, such as patientslikeme.com, offer good examples of the case in point.[8]

(2) The concept of *altruism* is well-established and should include data donation for the common good.[9] There is evidence that most individuals already desire

---

[6] This approach is clearly associated with some trade-offs, such as the creation of a dataset that is biased in favour of individuals who are willing to donate. However, this is not as such an argument against the choice of focusing initially on those willing to donate, as it has the benefit of using these "low-hanging fruit" to grow a wider social acceptance of PMDD and thus increasing the willingness to donate data.

[7] For example, see: Wellcome Trust Monitor: Wave 3 (full report). https://wellcome.ac.uk/sites/default/files/monitor-wave3-full-wellcome-apr16.pdf (accessed Sept 21, 2017).

[8] See https://www.personalgenomes.org.uk/ and https://www.patientslikeme.com/

[9] In the present context, the concept is to be broadly understood, as it is of course difficult to ascertain whether an individual really is an *altruist*, or whether other motives are behind a choice to act ethically.

to act morally, and may do so without the need for further encouragement when provided with the right information, a straightforward procedure, and appropriate safeguards (Richardson and Hurwitz 1995). With regard to PMDD, the lack of regulatory guidance and practical possibilities of donating data hampers the moral agency of potential donors.

(3) *Fairness* is also crucial, as it ensures that burdens and benefits are shared across society. If one receives healthcare, it is only fair that one gives back. This is an infra-generational argument, since members of the current generation will be donating data for the benefit of others, much like they currently benefit from the contributions of previous generations to medical knowledge. Arguably, there is a moral obligation to participate in scientific research (Harris 2005).

(4) PMDD is an appeal to inter-generational solidarity, as future generations will benefit from past generations and will become more motivated to donate to future generations in turn. Recently, the notion of *solidarity* has experienced a revival as a framework to direct biomedicine beyond the dichotomy of personal benefit and the common good (Prainsack 2017). Such arguments suggest that there is a need to nudge less altruistic individuals to act more responsibly, and to take on their share of the collective burden of contributing to medical knowledge (Prainsack and Buyx 2017).

(5) PMDD would foster a (human) *right to science*. It has been argued that this includes a human right to participate in the scientific process in its entirety (Vayena and Tasioulas 2015). Of course, this is not to say that a right to donate one's medical record implies a receiver's duty to *use* these data, as it is advisable to retain the option to reject a donation where this carries significant ethical risks. This is standard practice in whole-body donation programmes, where acceptance of a donation is contingent on the health status of the donor and the demand by the accepting institution (Riederer et al. 2012).

(6) There is a strong *economic argument* to be made. Using the data that are already being collected during health and social care to advance the body of medical knowledge would enable a more cost-effective administration of healthcare. In addition, the more data are donated, the more value the old data have. This scale issue is typical of the digital, and makes it economically sensible to encourage PMDD.[10]

(7) It is crucial to facilitate PMDD immediately, as the trend towards *commercialisation* of personal health data is growing, and this may leave the public at risk of missing out. Public and commercial benefits are often intertwined, but there is a great risk that a lack of public systems that enable the donation of data may lead to the collection of such data occurring exclusively in the private/commercial sphere and that, consequently, the use of data for public benefit may become

[10] See the NHS Digital Business Plan 2017–2018. https://digital.nhs.uk/business-plan-2017-2018 (accessed March 5, 2018).

impossible, or at least restricted to research that has significant commercial value. Such a market is already emerging for individuals to sell their own data to companies. This is the case of Zenome.io, which combines blockchain technology and digital currency to allow individuals to sell their personal genomic information.[11] Soon, more comprehensive platforms might encourage individuals to sell their full electronic health records, as these become increasingly available to patients. A socio-political decision to take the initiative on PMDD is thus urgently needed to seize this opportunity and to avoid serious negative implications for public health research, once this will be locked out of an increasingly commercialised industry in personal medical data, or has to pay for access, in the absence of a public data donation scheme.

(8) PMDD is also a matter of *logical coherence*. Considering that (most) people can already donate their organs and blood, and that it is possible to extract substantial data from those donations, it is logically incoherent not to allow PMDD. Furthermore, implicitly, individuals are already allowed and often enabled to give away freely their personal data to private corporations, often for uncertain purposes, as the terms and conditions of many commercial platforms make clear.

(9) Two key *risks* are diminished in PMDD, as both consent and privacy are less troublesome where the data relate to a deceased as opposed to a living person. This would avoid or at least mitigate many of the problems currently arising in the context of data sharing, as PMDD poses significantly less pressure on individual privacy, ownership, and consent.

(10) Finally, *data sharing* by research institutions has been encouraged in recent years and is now considered part of good scientific conduct, as it fosters transparency, replicability of studies, and leads to efficient use of research data. Given that most of the reasons for scientific data sharing also apply to PMDD, a decision to promote one but not the other is logically and ethically inconsistent.

While other types of medical donation (such as tissue donation) have been the subject of extensive debate, resulting in ethical and governance frameworks and national schemes, this has yet to occur for medical data donation. At the same time, public relations campaigns are ongoing to promulgate the need to utilise health data wisely and ethically. The high-profile UK campaign "Understanding Patient Data", which is jointly funded by the Wellcome Trust, the Medical Research Council, the Department of Health and Social Care, the Economic and Social Research Council, and Public Health England, aims to "support discussions with the public, patients and healthcare professionals about uses of health and care data".[12] This is an unethical asymmetry, since the lack of opportunity for individuals to donate their PMRs

[11] Zenome – Your DNA is an asset. Zenome is a market. https://zenome.io/ (accessed Oct 31, 2017).

[12] Understanding Patient Data. http://understandingpatientdata.org.uk/ (accessed November 5, 2018).

prevents them from acting altruistically by donating their data for the common good, despite public funding invested in educating the public about the need to make such data accessible for research within the health service. Research into the harms of non-use of health data has concluded that these are hard to prove, but that there are significant consequences that need to be addressed in a move towards socially responsible reuse of data (Jones et al. 2017). In addition, the aforementioned study did not consider the social harm of preventing people from doing what they deem to be morally important. That this is a real concern was shown by some participants in a large biobank study in Norway, where the desire to contribute to the common good was frequently brought up (Steinsbekk et al. 2013). Once all this is combined with the potential value that such data hold for medical research, it provides a strong reason for remedying the current missed opportunity. The fact that the current lack of a mechanism for PMDD is more likely to be explained by regulatory inertia than a deliberate decision against it on ethical grounds provides even more reason to remedy the situation. So, how does PMDD compare to the existing types of biomedical donation that are already managed by specific ethical guidelines and governance frameworks? The next section addresses this question.

11.4 How Does PMDD Compare to Other Biomedical Donations?

A number of types of biomedical donation are already firmly established in several health systems around the world. Currently, there are at least seven types of physical donations, plus two where the donation consists of a specific data set. Given this abundance of donation schemes, one might question the need for yet another framework and suggest instead an ethical approach by analogy. However, as Table 11.2 indicates by focusing on the United Kingdom, there are some morally significant differences among existing schemes and the proposed PMDD.

11.4.1 Key Differences Among Existing Biomedical Donation Schemes

The first key difference between PMDD and the most common donation schemes is the lack of physical intrusion. Although donating medical data can be described as being intrusive to private life, it does not involve a physical act, or indeed any action on behalf of the donor other than giving consent. This is also a one-off task, as there is no opportunity for re-contact when the donor is deceased.

This leads to the second key difference: donor status. Blood, gametes, cord blood, and tissue are usually donated by living people, as are some organs (e.g. some kidneys). However, even where the donations are by the deceased, the living

Table 11.2 Comparison of biomedical donation schemes in the United Kingdom

Donation type	Donor status: Living (L), Deceased (D)	Physical (P), Digital (D)	Beneficiary: Self (S), Others (O)	Purpose: Medical (M), Research (R), Teaching (T), Art (A)	Benefit: Immediate (I), Variable (V), Undefined (U)	Governance scheme: National (N), Corporate (C), Institutional (I)	Commercial schemes (Yes, No)
Blood	L	P	S, O	M, R	I	N	N
Cord blood	L	P	S, O	M, R	U	N, C	Y
Gametes	L	P	S, O	M	V	N, C	Y
Tissue	L	P	O	R	V	N, I	N
Organs	D[a]	P	O	M	I	N	N
Brain	D	P	O	R	I	I	N
Bodies	D	P	O	R, T, A	I	I	Y[b]
Research participation	L	D	S, O	R	V	I	Y
Genome	L	D	S, O	R	V	I	Y
Data (PMD)	D*	D	O	R	U	I	Y

[a]Exceptions apply, such as kidney donations by living donors
[b]A rare example is the commercial art project "Body Worlds"
* This applies to the current proposal for posthumous donations, but this may be extended to living donors in the future

relatives are typically directly involved: organ donations are checked with family members prior to proceeding, and the urgency of the process (with arrangements typically made within 24 h of death) can put immense pressure on relatives. With PMDD, it might be equally sensible to bring family members on board, even where the deceased have clearly expressed their wishes, but no urgency is required as the utility of the data has no expiry date.

A third difference relates to the materiality of data: medical or any kind of digital data are non-material, unlike other biomedical donations. This means, for instance, that data cannot be "taken out" of one individual and put into another – as would be the case in organ or blood donations.

This is linked to a final difference worth stressing, namely that of the beneficiary. While blood, cord blood, and gamete donations can be used to benefit oneself in the future (although that might be more accurately described as a safeguard than a donation), with other donations, including PMDD, the beneficiaries are necessarily others. In addition, where the purpose of the donation is non-clinical there is no immediate benefit to anyone in particular. The benefit is of a more general nature, such as the advancement of clinical knowledge through research, or the teaching and training of future health care professionals. When it comes to donations that involve health or medical data, as opposed to a physical donation, the key difference lies in the research question. Typically, clinical research studies and trials will attempt to answer a specific question, or address a concrete hypothesis, whereas PMDD would be used for more general research and promote serendipity in research.[13] Researchers in traditional clinical studies will have to re-contact their participants if they wish to use the data for further or additional research, this requirement does not apply in PMDD. In addition, living participants can change their mind at any point and withdraw their consent, meaning that their data is removed from any research in so far as this is practically possible, which again does not apply in PMDD, where active consent management is an impossibility.

These differences listed above are only some of the most significant ones between existing forms of biomedical donation and PMDD. The list is by no means exhaustive. Yet, the comparison suffices to highlight that reliance on existing frameworks is likely to fall short of offering the ethical guidance required to enable safe PMDD. This is also because, although some important risks are minimised, PMDD is not without its own risks. These risks need to be carefully managed while maximising the future utility of the donated data. This makes it of utmost importance to ensure that PMDD is done ethically, and in particular safely and fairly, without creating any unnecessary impediment to either the donor or the health researcher using their data.

[13] With the exception of biobanks, where data are collected for a range of future research studies.

11.5 The Need for an Ethical Code

Broadly speaking, two main sources of risks can be associated with PMDD, one resulting from the non-individual nature of medical data and one resulting from source of the data being a deceased individual without any control over future uses of the data.

The first source concerns the *nature* of the donated medical data, specifically that medical data is seldom just about one individual but also often relates to others, who may be harmed as a result Some of the donor's medical data may reveal sensitive information about related people. Relational issues arise, for instance, where genomic data reveal information about family members. Similarly, information found in psychological or psychiatric records may well contain sensitive information about others, including family members, as this often plays a significant part in the treatment of mental illness. Sexual health and reproductive information are further examples of sensitive medical data that typically relate to at least one other person. Harms to others might also be caused when insights derived from donated data are used for profiling purposes, which might be discriminatory and unfair to individuals to whom it is applied. This risk becomes more acute when donated medical data is sensitive, for example when relating to a particular (other) individual or a sensitive condition. In some cases, the risks may be such to embargo a donation, or in extreme cases to disallow an individual from participating in PMDD, despite a personal desire to do so. An example could be close relatives of acting politicians, where there is a national interest in avoiding the exposure of vulnerabilities to outside influences. Similarly, some conditions, like hereditary diseases or mental illness, may carry a significantly greater risk of becoming a target of discrimination, making it preferable to avoid PMDD. The overall cost of this restriction would be minimal, as the value of PMDD lies in well-curated, large data sets, rather than individual data sets. It is important to understand that, when shared data pose a serious risk, it would be ethically justified and sensible to reject the particular data donation, as the limited value of a single data set (or even of a particularly valuable one), is outweighed by the risks to other, living members of society. The decision as to when to reject a donation should be strictly limited to those cases where the risk to others is likely and serious, to avoid that overcautiously approaches may lead to the dismissal of valuable data sets that could be useful to study less common conditions and rare diseases.

In summary, fears around potential harms to close relatives do not represent an argument against PMDD. The risks just highlighted are not specific to PMDD but rather refer to the *kind* of data in question, not the actual *act* of donating. This means that all the risks generally associated with biomedical data also apply in this context (Mittelstadt and Floridi 2016). The consequence is that one can rely on similar safeguards, especially in terms of the procedures, policies and tools that are already applied in the healthcare context, such as de-identification and encryption.[14] The fact that these data would be *donated* does not affect these concerns substantially.

The second source of risks concerns the provenance of the donated medical data and the potential use to which the donated data can be put. Because the donor is deceased, PMDD has a lower (or perhaps no) negative impact on the donor, compared with sharing one's medical data when alive. However, safeguarding is also lower, since individuals may indicate how their data may be used or repurposed while they are alive, but of course have no control once dead. It is therefore crucial to develop a framework that respects the values and preferences of the data donors, and that reassures potential donors that their expressed wishes will be respected after death. In particular, concerns over the misuse of medical Big Data to justify unfair public policies, the implementation of medical profiling outside of the health care context (e.g. by employers or insurance companies), and the application of IP rights to lock-in or restrict access to medical insights and advances derived from donated medical data have to be taken seriously, and need to be addressed.

For all these reasons, an ethical code of PMDD is needed to these issues effectively. With regard to the first risk (of harm to relatives), encouraging the active involvement of family members and relatives prior to a decision to participate in PMDD could resolve many of the potential concerns, similar to the existing recommendations in organ or body donation. As it has been argued, a "do not use if in doubt" approach is also practicable, as the value of any single data set is limited and unlikely to have an impact on the utility of the overall PMDD database. Note that this is also an argument against the need to impose a "duty to easy rescue", and hence a suspension of the need to have informed consent: one organ not donated may mean a life not saved, but one data set not included makes in itself little difference to population-based medical studies.

The second risk (lack of control once deceased) can be mitigated by means of a value-based framework that firmly places key ethical principles—such as respect for persons, human dignity, privacy and integrity, amongst others—at the heart of PMDD. Two valuable resources can be drawn on to inform such a code. First, the lessons learned from past mistakes made in the context of biomedical data schemes, such as the NHS Care.data programme, as well as the best practices of ongoing initiatives, such as the Personal Genome Project UK. And second, the ethical and governance frameworks currently in place for other types of donations, most crucially those used in biobanking, organ and body donation. An ethical code for PMDD must learn from the solutions already found for both these resources, and be coherent with them. In the next chapter, we set out to codify some of the lessons and best practices that currently exist in an unstructured form to develop a functional ethical code for PMDD, as well as leverage the important work done by others in developing ethical frameworks for other types of biomedical donations (see Chap. 12).

[14] For example, see the Wellcome Trust's 2013 "Summary report of qualitative research into public attitudes to personal data and linking personal data", available at: https://wellcomelibrary.org/item/b20997358#?c=0&m=0&s=0&cv=0

11.6 How to Implement Ethical PMDD

The first step towards the development of an ethical code for PMDD presented in this article was a thorough review of existing ethical frameworks. The focus was in particular on tissue, brain, and body donation, as well as the sharing of genomic information, because of their similarities with PMDD. However, our analysis also revealed some key differences (discussed above), limiting direct comparability with our proposed scheme, and reinforcing our belief that a dedicated code is needed for PMDD. In this section, some past and current biomedical data projects are considered to identify relevant lessons and best practice.

11.6.1 Learning from Mistakes and Codifying Best Practice

Big Data in health care is often described as the biggest opportunity of our times to improve public and individual health, and it is therefore no surprise that a vast number of data-related projects are ongoing in health care. While there are key differences among the initiatives, including in data ownership, access rights and purpose, their success—in terms of ethics—can be evaluated on the basis of adherence to a number of fundamental principles.

At the unsuccessful end of the spectrum, initiatives like the UK's disastrous Care.data serve as a reminder that neglecting these principles can lead to the complete failure of a well-intended scheme. As the Nuffield Council on Bioethics has explained, "Care.data is a salutary lesson in the need for robust and timely public engagement – as opposed to mere communication – and in understanding the range of ways in which data subjects might perceive harms arising from uses of their data."[15] The consequences of this incident can still be felt, and have led to a deep distrust in data sharing between the NHS and commercial partners. This is in contrast with other countries, where better management of communication and public engagement has led to wide public support of similar programmes (Patil et al. 2016).

Unfortunately, it seems that some of the lessons learnt from the Care.data debacle have not yet been applied. The recent introduction of the "GP at hand" video-consultation smartphone app, for which NHS England partnered with Babylon Health, has met with skepticism both from GPs and the general public. Concerns quickly arose over inequality in the treatment of patients, especially those with complex health needs, ultimately leading to a suspension of the planned wider roll-out of the service (Finlayson et al. 2017). The lack of proper evaluation of the service has also been criticised (Rosen 2017), and concerns raised over the privacy management, given Babylon Health assumes ownership of the recorded video

[15] See: Laurie et al. (2014) "A review of evidence relating to harm resulting from uses of health and biomedical data" available at https://nuffieldbioethics.org/wp-content/uploads/FINAL-Report-on-Harms-Arising-from-Use-of-Health-and-Biomedical-Data-30-JUNE-2014.pdf

consultations in its terms and conditions.[16] Although this might seem unlikely to be enforced in practice, in theory this means that patients are not allowed to share their video consultations with health care professionals who are not enrolled with Babylon's GP at hand service without the company's prior permission. Considering that the service was commissioned by NHS England, most patients are likely to be unaware of this restriction, and hiding such an important point in the legal text does not exemplify good communication or foster trust between the NHS, its third-party partners, and patients.

In the context of genetic data, the Icelandic genetic testing company, deCODE Genetics, provides another example of how public trust is all too easily disappointed. In 2012, the company decided to sell out to the American pharmaceutical company Amgen—including the DNA and health data of approximately 140,000 Icelandic individuals held by deCODE. Most of these people had volunteered their data on the basis that the company would create a universal health database of Icelanders for research purposes, as it had promised in the late 1990s but never delivered (Greely 2012).

Sustainability is crucial for any health-related Big Data project, as its success will depend on a long-term commitment to research. Unfortunately, this aspect is often neglected. A few years ago, the Finnish government (in cooperation with some private sector companies) launched the ambitious project of setting up a single platform for the storage of information on the health and well-being of the population. The idea was that this could be accessed by health care providers to offer more efficient and effective care, and to prevent ill health. The service, taltioni.fi, was lauded as sustainable and trustworthy, not least because of its cooperative nature and the fact that it involved both the public and private sectors (Riso et al. 2017). However, the platform vanished shortly after its launch, and it is not known what happened to any data stored within it.[17]

At the other end of the spectrum are projects like the "Patients Like Me" network, which according to its website, is "unleashing the power of data for good (…) by empowering people to take control of their health."[18] The company provides a detailed and clear privacy policy, including plain language explanations in addition to legal texts, and provides users with comprehensive options to manage the sharing of their data with third parties, such as private corporations and commercial vendors.

The Personal Genome Project UK (PGP-UK) is equally transparent about data access, but goes one step further by providing the de-identified genomic information as fully Open Data. Individuals can choose to withdraw their data at any point but are made aware, before enrolment, that such a withdrawal cannot necessarily prevent all future uses of the data, as copies of it may have been downloaded from the website. The PGP-UK is complex in that it involves sharing of genomic data as

---

[16] See: https://web.archive.org/web/20171114123501/https://www.gpathand.nhs.uk/legal/terms (accessed March 5, 2018).

[17] As reported by the Finnish Data Protection Office: http://www.tietosuoja.fi/fi/index/blogi/6IUtCELFH/2017/XHtWkkNPr.html.stx (accessed March 5, 2018).

[18] See: https://www.patientslikeme.com/about

Open Data, and this is reflected in the informed consent procedure, which requires participants to pass an enrolment exam before being admitted to the project.

Even a deep commitment to ethical principles offers no guarantee that things will never go wrong, as accidental breaches are always possible. In 2014, the PGP suffered a setback when it accidentally disclosed some of the participant email addresses and names to other participants.[19] Due to a configuration error, replies to an email from the PGP-UK were sent to the entire mailing list rather than the PGP-UK staff only, thereby revealing the sender's identity to the members of the list. Some 220 people were affected, and the issue was quickly discussed within the ethics community, where it was described as a failure both in privacy and trust.[20] This is just one interpretation, as the PGP-UK notified and apologised immediately after the event, but the incident indicated that risk from human error is hard to eliminate. As one of the commentators in the discussion noted, the email blunder was a suitable way to identify those prospective participants who merely pay lip service to the idea of openly sharing their data.

Recently, cooperative models for managing personal health data have gained popularity. Switzerland currently has two such schemes, healthbank and MIDATA. Both enable citizens to be in control of the storage, management and access of their personal health and health-related data, including the decision how to share it. Schemes like these find their inspiration in citizen science, whereby members of the public can contribute actively to medical research by providing access to their personal data. As these platforms are fairly recent developments and are not yet in place in most countries, it remains to be seen how they will be adopted by the public. However, their cooperative approach certainly carries great potential for the future management of personal health data.

11.6.2 Deriving Relevant Ethical Principles

Drawing on the review of the literature and relevant biomedical donation schemes and projects, and the input from the participants of two workshops on the ethics of data donation,[21] the following five ethical principles or categories emerged as most relevant to PMDD:

---

[19] See: https://www.personalgenomes.org.uk/archive/email-storm-incident-and-apology (accessed March 5, 2018).

[20] See, for example, Boddington (2014) "Personal Genome Project UK email disaster: If you can't guarantee privacy, at least try to ensure trust", available at: http://blog.practicalethics.ox.ac.uk/2014/05/personal-genome-project-uk-email-disaster-if-you-cant-guarantee-privacy-at-least-try-to-ensure-trust/ (accessed March 5, 2018).

[21] Two workshops on the ethics of medical data donation were held in Oxford in October 2017 and April 2018, which included experts from academia, policy-making and industry. In addition to common principles from the academic literature, valuable points from practice were shared and contributed to the identification of key ethical principles for PMDD. The workshops were supported by a research grant from Microsoft Research.

1. Human dignity and respect for persons
2. Promotion of the common good
3. The right to "Citizen Science"
4. Quality and good data governance
5. Transparency, accountability, and integrity

These might at first glance appear rather generic and hardly ground-breaking. One might also question how these can be applied in practice. In response, we lay out the specific requirements for an "Ethical Code for Posthumous Data Donation" in the Appendix, which provides more detail on a practical implementation. The Code is not a governance framework, so some practical issues will still need to be addressed before implementing a PMDD scheme. With regard to the generality of the principles, this is crucial to preserve sufficient flexibility to account for future developments. Considering that PMDD is going to be a long-term endeavour, it is important to regulate for the future, i.e. to avoid ethical guidelines becoming inapplicable due to technological, legal, cultural or social changes. This is the goal of the Code proposed here: to provide normative principles shaping PMDD, rather than a set of specific rules of conduct for the involved actors. These are not based on any singular ethical approach (such as a consequentialist ethics) but build on human rights, the concept of human dignity and bioethical principles, including research ethical principles.

11.7 Conclusion

In light of both the benefits and potential risks involved in wide donation of personal medical data, there is a need for an ethical code of PMDD that addresses key challenges, including consent, privacy, security and ownership. The previous work done in relation to other types of biomedical donation acts as a useful resource to inform such a code but cannot simply be extended to PMDD, which comes with its own particular ethical challenges.

It is argued that most of these issues have practical solutions, and that the primary focus should be on managing permissible access and use of the collected data. Procedural safeguards have already been developed in other relevant and comparable areas of medical research and could be adopted to foster PMDD. Consider for example the broad consent procedures currently used in biobanking or the "educate-before-you-sign" approach similar to the one used by the PGP-UK. This would ensure that any individual wishing to donate medical data could make a decision that is maximally informed (Sheehan 2011). Privacy risks could be mitigated by managing carefully access to donated data. At the same time, it is important to emphasise that no safety measures will ever be fail-safe, and openness about this fact should form part of the ethical design of PMDD procedures.

The code developed here (see the following chapter) addresses the key ethical issues arising from PMDD. Arguably, before being adopted, further input should be obtained from a wider audience, for instance through public engagement, to investigate public support. However, this is only the first step towards more comprehensive use of health-relevant data for the common good. In the future, combining corporate data (via data philanthropy) with data sharing and PMDD might open up even greater possibilities for supporting health care and research. But for this to work, PMDD must first be brought to life.

References

Boddington, P. 2014. Personal genome project UK email disaster: If you can't guarantee privacy, at least try to ensure trust - Practical Ethics blog, University of Oxford. http://blog.practicalethics.ox.ac.uk/2014/05/personal-genome-project-uk-email-disaster-if-you-cant-guarantee-privacy-at-least-tryto-ensure-trust/. Accessed 5 Nov 2018.

Finlayson, A.E., E. Barry, L. Craven, and T. Greenhalgh 2017. Primary healthcare, disruptive innovation, and the digital gold rush. *The BMJ*. http://blogs.bmj.com/bmj/2017/11/21/primary-healthcare-disruptive-innovation-and-the-digital-gold-rush. Accessed 5 Mar 2018.

Floridi, L., and P. Illari. 2016. *The philosophy of information quality*. Cham: Springer.

Greely, H. 2012. *Amgen buys DeCODE – reflections backwards, forwards, and on DTC genomics*. Stanford Law School. https://law.stanford.edu/2012/12/13/lawandbiosciences-2012-12-13-amgen-buys-decode-reflections-backwards-forwards-and-on-dtc-genomics. Accessed Mar 5 2018.

Haeusermann, T., B. Greshake, A. Blasimme, D. Irdam, M. Richards, and E. Vayena. 2017. Open sharing of genomic data: Who does it and why? *PLoS One* 12: e0177158.

Harris, J. 2005. Scientific research is a moral duty. *Journal of Medical Ethics* 31: 242–248.

Jones, K.H., G. Laurie, L. Stevens, C. Dobbs, D.V. Ford, and N. Lea. 2017. The other side of the coin: Harm due to the non-use of health-related data. *International Journal of Medical Informatics* 97: 43–51.

Laurie, G., K.H. Jones, L. Stevens, and C. Dobbs. 2014. A review of evidence relating to harm resulting from uses of health and biomedical data. *Nuffield Council on Bioethics*.

Mann, S.P., J. Savulescu, and B.J. Sahakian. 2016. Facilitating the ethical use of health data for the benefit of society: Electronic health records, consent and the duty of easy rescue. *Philosophical Transactions of the Royal Society A: Mathematical, Physical and Engineering Sciences* 374: 20160130.

Mittelstadt, B.D., and L. Floridi. 2016. *The ethics of biomedical big data*. Cham: Springer.

Patil, S., H. Lu, C.L. Saunders, D. Potoglou, and N. Robinson. 2016. Public preferences for electronic health data storage, access, and sharing—Evidence from a pan-European survey. *Journal of the American Medical Informatics Association* 23: 1096–1106.

Prainsack, B. 2015. Why we should stop talking about data sharing. *DNAdigest*. http://dnadigest.org/why-we-should-stop-talking-about-data-sharing/. Accessed 20 July 2018.

———. 2017. The "We" in the "Me": Solidarity and health care in the era of personalized medicine. *Science Technology and Human Values* 43: 21–44.

———. 2018. Data donation: How to resist the iLeviathan. In *The ethics of medical data donation*, ed. J. Krutzinna and L. Floridi. Springer.

Prainsack, B., and A. Buyx. 2017. *Solidarity in biomedicine and beyond*. Cambridge: Cambridge University Press. https://doi.org/10.1017/9781139696593.

Richardson, R., and B. Hurwitz. 1995. Donors' attitudes towards body donation for dissection. *The Lancet* 346: 277–279.

Riederer, B.M., S.H. Bolt, E. Brenner, J.L. Bueno-López, A.R. Circulescu, D.C. Davies, R.D. Caro, P.O. Gerrits, S. McHanwell, D. Pais, and F. Paulsen. 2012. The legal and ethical framework governing body donation in Europe – 1st update on current practice. *European Journal of Anatomy* 16 (1): 1–21.

Riso, B., A. Tupasela, D.F. Vears, H. Felzmann, J. Cockbain, M. Loi, N.C. Kongsholm, S. Zullo, and V. Rakic. 2017. Ethical sharing of health data in online platforms – Which values should be considered? *Life Sciences, Society and Policy* 13: 12.

Rosen, R. 2017. Are disruptive innovators in GP provision strengthening or weakening the NHS? *BMJ* 359: j5470.

Shaw, D.M., J.V. Gross, and T.C. Erren. 2015. Data donation after death. *The Lancet* 386: 340.

———. 2016. Data donation after death. *EMBO Reports* 17: 14–17.

Sheehan, M. 2011. Can broad consent be informed consent? *Public Health Ethics* 4: 226–235.

Steinsbekk, K.S., L.Ø. Ursin, J.-A. Skolbekken, and B. Solberg. 2013. We're not in it for the money—Lay people's moral intuitions on commercial use of 'their' biobank. *Medicine, Health Care, and Philosophy* 16: 151–162.

Taddeo, M. 2016. Data philanthropy and the design of the infraethics for information societies. *Philosophical Transactions of the Royal Society A: Mathematical, Physical and Engineering Sciences* 374: 20160113.

Vayena, E., and J. Tasioulas. 2015. "We the scientists": A human right to citizen science. *Philosophy & Technology* 28: 479–485.

Chapter 12
An Ethical Code for Posthumous Medical Data Donation

Jenny Krutzinna, Mariarosaria Taddeo, and Luciano Floridi

Abstract This chapter follows the argument that personal medical data should be made available for scientific research by enabling and encouraging individuals to donate their medical records after death, provided that this can be done safely and ethically. While medical donation schemes with dedicated regulatory and ethical frameworks for blood, organ or tissue donations are already in place, no such ethical guidance currently exists with regard to personal medical data. In addressing this gap, this chapter presents the first ethical code for posthumous medical data donation (PMDD). It is based on five foundational principles and seeks to inform and guide the implementation of an effective and ethical PMDD scheme by addressing the key risks associated with the utilisation of personal health data for the promotion of the common good.

Keywords Data donation · Medical data ethics · Ethical code · Health records · Personal health data · Data philanthropy · Data ethics

12.1 Preamble

The importance and value of brain, body, organ and tissue donation after death has long been recognised, and relevant regulatory and ethical frameworks have been put in place to manage it. Medical data, which also hold enormous potential for medical research and for the improvement of health and social care on a large scale, has not as yet been incorporated into such frameworks. Neither is it currently possible to

J. Krutzinna (✉)
Department of Administration and Organization Theory, University of Bergen, Bergen, Norway
e-mail: jenny.krutzinna@uib.no

M. Taddeo · L. Floridi
Oxford Internet Institute, University of Oxford, Oxford, UK

The Alan Turing Institute, London, UK
e-mail: mariarosaria.taddeo@oii.ox.ac.uk; luciano.floridi@oii.ox.ac.uk

J. Krutzinna, L. Floridi (eds.), *The Ethics of Medical Data Donation*, Philosophical Studies Series 137, https://doi.org/10.1007/978-3-030-04363-6_12

donate one's medical data posthumously.[1] However, enabling such *posthumous medical data donation* (hereafter PMDD) is in the interest of individuals and society at large. It is important to make medical data available for scientific research by enabling and encouraging individuals to donate their medical records[2] after death, similarly to how they can already donate bodies or body parts. This is why a research project on PMDD, developed by the Digital Ethics Lab at the Oxford Internet Institute has led to the formulation of this Ethical Code for Posthumous Medical Data Donation (hereafter the Code), which sets out the guiding ethical principles for such donations. An important limitation to note is that the Code focuses exclusively on ethical aspects. This means that important practical issues relating to law and governance will have to be addressed prior to and during its implementation.[3]

12.2 Considerations

- Recalling the Convention for the Protection of Human Rights and Fundamental Freedoms of the Council of Europe, Rome, 4.XI.1950;
- Recalling the Convention on Human Rights and Biomedicine and the additional protocols to the Convention of the Council of Europe, Oviedo, 4.IV.1997;
- Recalling the Universal Declaration of Human Rights, 10.XII.1948 and the Universal Declaration on the Human Genome and Human Rights, 11.XI.1997 and the International Declaration on Human Genetic Data of the United Nations, 16.X.2003;
- Recalling the Universal Declaration of Bioethical Principles of the United Nations 19.X.2005;
- Recalling the Declaration of Helsinki of the World Medical Association, 1. VI.1964;
- Recalling the Regulation (EU) 2016/679 of the European Parliament and of the Council of 27 April 2016 on the protection of natural persons with regard to the processing of personal data and on the free movement of such data (GDPR), and repealing Directive 95/46/EC.

[1] Arguably, there are no particular barriers to donate one's data, at least in some jurisdictions such as the UK, where this could be done via an Advance Directive. However, the lack of coherent ethical and legal structure to facilitate such donation makes it practically impossible.

[2] The term "medical records"is to be loosely understood, as the availability and format will vary between jurisdictions and it is unlikely that medical data are consolidated in one place.

[3] See the concept of post-compliance soft ethics in Floridi, L. 2018. Soft ethics, the governance of the digital and the general data protection regulation. Philosophical Transactions of the Royal Society A 376 (2133): 20180081.

12.3 Definitions

Term	Definition
Commercial exploitation	The sale, lease or commercial licensing of the data. It shall also include uses of the data to produce or manufacture products or services for general sale.
Donor	The person-source of the data, or data subject.
Data	Any donor-related data.
Database	Repository (often online) built to facilitate access to data.
Directly identifying data	Any data that make possible the identification of the person concerned, without disproportionate efforts.
De-anonymised / pseudo-anonymised / coded data	Any data that make possible the identification of the person concerned only through the use of a simple tool, such as a key.
Fully-anonymised data	Any data that do not make possible the identification of the person concerned without disproportionate efforts.
Information on hereditary disease	Any data which is either predictive of genetic disease or can serve to identify the person as a carrier of a gene responsible for a disease or detect a genetic predisposition or susceptibility to a disease, whereas scientific proof for validity of that information is present.
Informed consent	Informed, free and express decision to donate one's PMR after death for research purposes.
Personal Medical Record (PMR)	The health data stored about a person within the health system.
Posthumous Medical Data Donation (PMDD)	The giving of one's PMR for research purposes upon death.
PMDD activities	Activities such as obtaining, handling, processing, storing and distributing of data, including all associated research activities.
PMDD institution (PMDDI)	The PMDDI is the institutional body acting as steward of all donated data.
Researcher	Any person with a legitimate interest in conducting research, whether affiliated with an academic, commercial, public, private or other institution. It shall not include private individuals.
Steward	Institution holding and maintaining the data. The steward assumes full responsibility for compliance with the legal and ethical rules that apply to collecting, processing and managing the data.
User	Any person involved in collecting, storing, handling, processing, accessing, or managing the data.

12.4 Overview

The Code of Ethics on Posthumous Medical Data Donation (hereafter 'the Code') has been developed to establish the guiding ethical principles for Posthumous Medical Data Donation (hereafter 'PMDD'), in recognition that PMDD constitutes an act that is both meaningful to an individual and valuable to the public and as such should be facilitated.

12.4.1 Objectives

The key objective of the Code is to state the fundamental *ethical* principles which should govern all PMDD activities. In addition,

- any applicable national laws or local regulations are to be complied with at all times. The Code does not replicate, amend or overrule but complements any such instruments;[4]
- participation in PMDD activities is and remains voluntary; this includes every person's right to accept or refuse participation at any point;
- the autonomy and confidentiality of all donors and their families shall be respected;
- special care will be taken in all PMDD activities to avoid discrimination against, or stigmatisation of, an individual, a family or a group;
- every care will be taken that the collected data is used, and in line with the purposes for which it was donated, namely for ethically and scientifically sound research, and that it is not abandoned;
- the research process and the ethical guidelines will be reviewed by an independent body on a regular basis to take into account any new developments in technology, law, and society. The results of such a review will be made public.

12.4.2 Scope

The Code shall apply to the full range of PMDD activities involving donated personal medical records (hereafter 'PMR'). It shall not apply to other types of health-related data, nor shall it apply to donations made by living donors. For the purposes of the Code, PMDD shall not include donations made to private institutions for the purposes of commercial exploitation. The Code shall apply to donors, users, and researchers.

12.5 Foundational Ethical Principles

Five foundational principles aim to guarantee a minimum ethical standard to be maintained in all PMDD activities:

1. Human dignity and respect for persons
2. Promotion of the common good
3. The right to Citizen Science

[4]The Code presupposes some basic data protection and privacy safeguards in line with the legal instruments set out under "Considerations" above. This means that the Code may not be sufficiently detailed in jurisdictions that do not subscribe to those international conventions, and further guidelines may be required.

4. Quality and good data governance
5. Transparency, accountability, and integrity

12.5.1 Human Dignity and Respect for Persons

Human dignity and respect for persons shall be paramount in all PMDD activities. In particular,

- the dignity of the donor shall be protected at all times;
- the preferences and values of the donor shall be honoured at all times;
- the privacy of the donor shall be maintained;
- potential harm to the donor, any relatives and/or next of kin shall be minimised.

12.5.2 Promotion of the Common Good

The purpose of the PMDD database is to provide the means to generate and disseminate new medical knowledge to benefit the public. The donor's wish to promote the common good by contributing to biomedical research shall be respected. This means:

- to maximise the morally good outcome, all PMDD shall be publicly accessible, and all research findings and results based on the data shall be published under an open licence;
- where the acceptance of a donation to the database carries a significant risk to relatives and/or family members, a careful balancing of harms and benefits should take place, which may lead to the rejection of the donation. Such rejections should be limited to serious cases of harm, to reduce the risk of excluding particularly valuable datasets, such as those relating to rare diseases and less common conditions. In all instances, the relatives and family members of the donor should be engaged in the process as much as is practically feasible to gain their support for the donation;
- prohibition of unethical research using PMDD without exception;
- prohibition of commercial exploitation of PMDD data where this could unfairly restrict access to treatments or cures;
- requesting proof of adequate benefit sharing measures prior to granting access to the PMDD database to a researcher.

12.5.3 The Right to Citizen Science

Citizens' right to participate in the scientific process in its entirety should be recognised and respected at all times. In particular,

- all donations should be accepted, unless there are solid grounds for rejecting a particular donation, such as a disproportionate risk of harm to others;
- the optimal use of donated data shall be guaranteed, and data shall not be abandoned;
- all results and findings shall be shared with the public in an accessible and timely manner;
- the public shall be actively involved in the further development of PMDD and encouraged to participate in deliberations about the wider social impact of PMDD.

12.5.4 Quality and Good Data Governance

Quality management and data governance shall be taken seriously when accepting, handling or using PMDD data. In particular,

- users and other PMDDI staff shall be adequately trained for their respective roles within the PMDD activities, including knowledge and understanding of this Code and any applicable data protection and privacy laws and regulations (such as the EU's General Data Protection Regulation);
- safe and secure storage facilities shall be used for the data, including use of adequate and updated encryption techniques, to minimise the risk of unauthorised access, data loss, or misuse. Proper record-keeping and access management shall be maintained to ensure full traceability of the location of, and access to, any PMDD;
- PMDDs shall be de-identified using currently available standards, and re-identification shall be prohibited. Quality control mechanisms for PMRs shall be applied prior to data being added to the database;
- mechanisms should be adopted for ensuring the sustainability of the database for future use, including procedures to be followed in case of discontinuance of the PMDDI.

12.5.5 Transparency, Trust, and Integrity

Transparency, trust, and integrity shall inform all PMDD activities, including communications with the donor and the public. In particular,

- communications with donors, any relatives or next of kin, and the public shall be open, honest, clear, and objective. Any information provided shall be comprehensible to a non-expert person and shall be accessible;
- clear and transparent procedures for deciding requests for data access shall be established and made public, and shall apply equally to all researchers regardless

of their affiliation. All access requests, whether granted or declined, shall be made public;

- mechanisms to ensure accountability and to handle complaints shall be implemented, including mechanisms for identifying, reporting and managing incidents such as breaches, losses of data, or unauthorised access. Any incident shall be followed by rigorous investigation, and corresponding sanctions shall be instituted. In addition, procedures for handling lawful requests from law enforcement agencies shall be established;
- full disclosure of any financial arrangements involving PMDD data or financial gains derived from PMDD activities will be made.

12.6 Obtaining PMRs for Research Purposes

PMR shall be obtained and used for research purposes in accordance with applicable national laws and local regulations, and the principles set forth in the Code.

Due to the anticipated benefit to be derived from the research to be conducted using the data, resources shall be dedicated to encourage participation in PMDD. In particular, information shall be provided to the public to encourage donations, while at the same time safeguarding the voluntariness of participation.

Consent shall be required for all collections of PMDD and for the use of PMDD for biomedical research purposes, even where local laws do not require such authorisation. As part of the consent procedure, participation will be explained as an opportunity to contribute in the long term to the improvement of other people's health. Broad consent to research falling within the guidelines of this Code shall be deemed sufficient, as it is not possible to anticipate all ethically and scientifically sound future research uses.

12.6.1 Obtaining Consent

Prior to giving informed consent, the person concerned shall be offered appropriate information about the nature and purpose of PMDD, including examples of the type of research for which it will be used, the financial interests of the data collecting entity, and the management of access to and use of the data, including the kinds of safeguards that will be maintained.

Donors shall be informed that the full PMRs will be transferred to the PMDDI, including identifying information, to enable linkage between different datasets which is necessary to ensure maximum scientific utility of the overall database. However, donors shall be free to place restrictions on the use of their data and to exclude subsets of data from their donations. These preferences shall be recorded in the PMR in full. Donors shall be informed of their right to make changes to their preferences or to withdraw consent at any point prior to their death.

Donors shall be encouraged to discuss their decision with their relatives, especially those with close genetic links.

Donors shall be informed that the use of their PMDD is not guaranteed and that in some rare instances a particular PMDD may be rejected if it poses a significant risk of harm to an individual or a group. Information shall be provided on possible reasons for exclusion.

Consent shall be appropriately documented in the PMR and at the PMDDI.

12.6.2 *Persons Unable to Give Consent*

To avoid the exclusion of vulnerable populations from benefiting from the scientific advances resulting from large-scale biomedical research, and to ensure their representation within the data underlying such research, an active effort shall be made to include PMRs from all groups.

Where an individual is permanently unable to provide consent, due to a lack of legal capacity, the registration of a donor and subsequent donation may be carried out with the authorisation of the person's legal representative or guardian. The individual concerned shall be involved in the decision-making process as far as possible.

Similarly, where a minor is concerned, the parents or legal guardian shall be permitted to authorise a donation. The opinion of the minor shall be taken into consideration in proportion to the age and degree of maturity of the child.

Where an individual is temporarily unable to provide consent, due to a lack of legal capacity, registration as a donor shall be held off until capacity to consent is regained or a permanent incapacity has been confirmed by the medical professional.

12.6.3 *Changing or Withdrawing Consent*

Donors can withdraw consent for participation in PMDD at any time by submitting a revised authorisation form, or by notifying a health care professional. The objection will be recorded in the PMR and will ensure that data is not submitted to the PMDD database on the donor's death.

It shall also be possible for a person to record an objection to PMDD in their PMR.

A decision to object to PMDD, or to change or withdraw consent once given, shall not have a negative impact on the medical treatment or care of the person or lead to discrimination against that person.

Where a legal representative or guardian gave the authorisation for PMDD, the right to change or withdraw consent remains with that person for as long as they shall have legal guardianship of that person.

12.6.4 Refusing Donations

There may be ethical reasons for excluding a particular PMDD donation, which may be grounded, *inter alia*, in the nature or the source of data. The following list is not exhaustive, and there may be other grounds on which a PMDDI may decide to refuse to accept a PMDD.

The right of a PMDDI to refuse a PMDD shall be maintained, as the overall cost of these refusals would be minimal, since the value lies in well-curated, large datasets, rather than individual datasets.

12.6.4.1 Refusing a PMDD on Grounds of the Data's Nature

Where the donor's data may reveal sensitive data about related people, a stewarding PMDDI may decide to refuse a PMDD. In particular, where genomic data reveal information about family members, it may be preferable to exclude such data from the donation where a comprehensive risk assessment reveals an unacceptably high risk to living people. This may apply especially where the relatives are vulnerable people and/or the condition is a hereditary disease, which may lead to stigma and/or discrimination.

12.6.4.2 Refusing a PMDD on Grounds of the Data Source

In some rare cases, there may be reasons to reject a PMDD on the basis of its source. This means disallowing a particular individual from participating in PMDD, where a donation would carry a disproportionate risk to others. An example could be close relatives of acting politicians or diplomats, where there is a national interest in avoiding the exposure of vulnerabilities to outside influences.

12.6.4.3 Other Grounds for Refusing a PMDD

An institution may refuse to accept a particular PMDD on other grounds, including, for example, the potentially illegal nature of the collected data, but any reasons should be made sufficiently clear to the potential donor.

12.7 Research Approval, Conduct and Oversight

In accordance with the foundational principles of the Code, it will be fundamental for the success of the PMDD activities that public trust is maintained. For this, it is crucial to manage research activities carefully, by maintaining transparency and ensuring accountability of any individual involved.

12.7.1 General Principles

12.7.1.1 Prohibition of Financial Gain[5]

It shall be prohibited to gain financially from PMDD. Therefore, donors will not be offered any financial or other inducement to participate in PMDD. Since participation does not entail any expense for the donor, the issue of reimbursement does not arise.

The PMDDI shall not be permitted to sell data obtained from PMDD activities, or to make a profit from such activities. Any profits resulting from the charging of access or licencing fees have to reinvested in the maintenance and improvement of the PMDD database. The sole purpose of any fee shall be to support the financing of costs, maintenance and improvement of the PMDD database, and shall not be used to make profits.

12.7.1.2 Confidentiality[6]

All data in relation to donors and their families shall be collected, processed and used in accordance with the principle of confidentiality and the right to respect for private life.

The steward will ensure that data are anonymised, linked, and stored to the highest standards of security. Researchers will only be given access to anonymised data.

All users and staff handling the data will receive appropriate training for maintaining confidentiality and adherence with all relevant legislation.

Systems for data security and storage will be kept up to date and will be of the highest technical standard.

---

[5] It is important to note that the research in this article has focused exclusively on the ethical issues of PMDD, which means that governance questions have not been answered. This includes the question of the legal nature of the institutional body (the PMDDI), which will need to be addressed prior the implementation of a PMDD scheme.

[6] These technical issues will need to be addressed more fully prior to the implementation of a PMDD scheme. Maintaining confidentiality through anonymization will have to be reconciled with the need to retain an option for re-identification for quality management purposes. The Code follows current practices in other types of medical donation schemes, e.g. biobanking, where anonymized data is made available to researchers and identifying data is kept separate and is not made available for research.

12.7.1.3 Data Custody

Custody of the data will be transferred to the PMDDI upon the donor's death. This conveys a range of rights to the stewarding institution, in particular the right to take legal action against unauthorised use or abuse of the data. Donors will not have property rights in the data.

The PMDDI will not exercise their right to sell the data to third parties but will act as steward of the database, maintaining and developing it for the common good in accordance with its purpose.

This does not affect the right of the donor to give away, sell, or donate data to other parties.

12.7.1.4 Data Protection

All data will be collected, stored and handled in accordance with applicable data protection laws and regulations to safeguard the integrity of all data, e.g. in compliance with the EU's General Data Protection Regulation.

12.7.1.5 Directly Identifiable Data

Directly identifiable data, which will necessarily be included in the transfer of the PMR to the PMDDI, will be separated from the medical data of the donor prior to being added to the database. An arbitrary code without any external meaning (that is, for example, not a National Insurance number or similar) will be attached to link the personal identifying information to the medical information. This option for re-identification is necessary for data quality management: to eliminate redundant data, verify data accuracy and completeness, to establish correct linkages among databases, and to identify data which may need to be withdrawn.

Identifying information will be held in a separate data vault with restricted access, controlled by a senior steward at the PMDDI. The access key to the code for re-linking identifying information to the data will never be shared with external agents, such as researchers, and will only be accessible to a select few PMDDI staff who are ethically trained and sign special confidentiality agreements.

12.7.1.6 Information on Health and Hereditary Disease

The PMDDI will not share data or health information with living relatives or other interested parties under any circumstances. This includes information on potential hereditary disease.

It is, however, possible for the donor to nominate specific individuals who are to receive a copy of the PMR upon the donor's death. It is the responsibility of the donor to ensure that the contact details of the recipients are kept up to date.

12.7.2 Research Access

The PMDDI will retain full control of all access to, and uses of, the data in the database. No exclusive access will be granted to any party.

To build and maintain a relationship of public trust, the PMDDI will inform the public of the rules for access, any requests made, access granted or refused, and any research results.

Access to the database by law enforcement agencies will be granted only under court order, and will be resisted in all other circumstances. Any such requests will be reported to the public in so far as this is legally permissible (see also clause 12.7.2.1).

The PMDDI may charge a reasonable fee for access to the data for approved research purposes. This fee may vary depending on the expected financial benefit from use of the data. However, the fee should not be so excessive as to prevent legitimate research from being conducted due to purely economic reasons, and it may in some circumstances be advisable to waive the fee entirely. Any profit occurring as a result of the fee system is regulated by clause 12.7.1.1.

12.7.2.1 Access Requests

The PMDDI will have overall decision-making authority over any access requests to the database. A special advisory board may be set up and charged with this task. However, routine applications may be delegated to appropriate working groups to provide more efficient services to the research community and to the public.

The PMDDI will provide public explanations of all policies and procedures for research access. These documents will continue to be developed to reflect relevant technical, legal and social changes, but will never abandon the principles of fairness and transparency in decision-making.

Access to the data will be granted only for scientifically and ethically approved research. Requestors will have to demonstrate benefit-sharing mechanisms and will have to have obtained research ethics approval from an appropriate body prior to being granted access to the data.

12.7.2.2 Research Results

All researchers accessing the database will be required to provide the results from their analyses made using the data, and any relevant supporting information, to the PMDDI to make them subsequently available to all other legitimate researchers with approved access to the database.

It is a requirement on all researchers seeking access to place the findings, whether positive or negative, from all research based on the PMDD data in the public domain. Publication of results shall be in peer-reviewed scientific literature wherever this is possible, open access by preference, or on the website of the PMDDI.

12.7.3 Research Oversight

Any PMDD activities will be conducted in accordance with national research governance frameworks and national research guidelines.

Independent periodic reviews of the quantity and quality of access requests, the research conducted, and the published results will be conducted and the findings will be made public.

As the purpose of PMDD is to generate new knowledge to promote population health, particular focus shall be placed on the dissemination of research outcomes. Where the independent reviewers are not satisfied that the principles of the Code are sufficiently upheld by the researchers, the PMDDI shall be required to review its access procedures to ensure that only those research requests are granted that promise to honour the principles of the Code.

12.7.4 Contingency Planning

The PMDDI shall develop a detailed contingency strategy for handling the PMDDI data and database in case of liquidation or termination of the PMDDI. The goal of the strategy must be to ensure the continuous protection of the rights of the donors and their families, and to respect their wishes that their data be used for research purposes. As such, the strategy should provide detailed plans for transferring the data to another steward so that research may continue on the data.

Annex: Sample PMDD Authorisation Form

To be completed by donor and signed by a witness.
Please complete in BLOCK CAPITALS

Title
Surname/family name
Forename(s)
Address
Tel no
Email
Date of birth

I WISH TO DONATE MY MEDICAL DATA AFTER MY DEATH.
I UNDERSTAND THAT THEY MAY BE USED FOR RESEARCH PURPOSES.

Please read the "Notes on completing these forms" then tick as appropriate

1. Data retention

☐ I consent to my medical data being retained indefinitely.
OR
☐ My medical data can be retained for a maximum of ___ years.

2. Data types

☐ I consent to all my medical data being used.
OR
☐ I wish to exclude the following data from my donation:

____

3. Research purposes

☐ I consent to my medical data being used for all research that has received ethics approval by an official REC within the European Economic Area (EU, plus Iceland, Liechtenstein and Norway).

4. Copy of record

☐ I wish the following named individuals to receive a complete copy of my medical data upon my death:

Name
Contact details

Witness details
Full Name
Address
Relationship to donor
Signatures
Date, Signature of donor
Date, Signature of witness

Acknowledgments We express our gratitude to Microsoft Research, for funding the research that led to the elaboration of this document. We are also extremely grateful to the participants of two workshops on the Ethics of Data Donation, held by the Digital Ethics Lab at the Oxford Internet Institute, for their valuable contribution to the preparation of this document.

Funded by Microsoft Research. The authors declare no conflict of interest.

References[7]

BrainNet Europe Code of Conduct by the BNE Consortium. 2008, May. Available at http://www.brainnet-europe.org/images/content/en/media/code/code_of_conduct.pdf.

Framework for responsible sharing of genomic and health-related data by the Global Alliance for Genomics and Health. 2014. Available at https://www.ga4gh.org/docs/ga4ghtoolkit/rsgh/Framework-Version-10September2014.pdf.

Human Tissue Authority's Code A: Guiding principles and the fundamental principle of consent, available at https://www.hta.gov.uk/sites/default/files/HTA%20%2807a-17%29%20Guiding%20Principles.pdf.

Overview of legal and ethical frameworks governing body donation in Europe by Riederer et al. 2016. Available at http://repository.ubn.ru.nl/bitstream/handle/2066/116823/116823.pdf?sequence=1.

UK Biobank Ethics and Governance Framework. Version 3.0, October 2007. Available at http://www.ukbiobank.ac.uk/wp-content/uploads/2011/05/EGF20082.pdf?phpMyAdmin=trmKQlYdjjnQIgJ%2CfAzikMhEnx6.

[7]This document draws heavily on the excellent ethical frameworks prepared by various organisations for other biomedical purposes, including the references under the heading "References".

Index

J. Krutzinna, L. Floridi (eds.), *The Ethics of Medical Data Donation*, Philosophical Studies Series 137, https://doi.org/10.1007/978-3-030-04363-6

www.ingramcontent.com/pod-product-compliance
Lightning Source LLC
LaVergne TN
LVHW082233200926
848484LV00008B/2347